THE CLINICIAN'S GUIDE TO PROFESSIONAL BOUNDARIES
What you don't know can end your career.

By Stephen Schenthal, MD, MSW Founder and CEO of PBI Education

ABOUT THE AUTHOR

Trained in both psychiatry and social work, Stephen Schenthal, MD, MSW had a successful private psychiatric practice for many years. Then, in 1999, he committed a professional boundary violation that ended his clinical career. As he journeyed through a civil suit, criminal prosecution, and ultimately the permanent revocation of his medical license, he continued to ask himself how he could have done such a thing. How does a decent person and a good doctor, who has devoted his life to healing others, commit an unethical and illegal act that harms his patients, family, friends, and profession?

After struggling through this intense period of introspection, research, and discussion with leading experts in the field, Dr. Schenthal created the PBI Violation Potential Formula© to define a professional's violation potential at any given time. Determined to help other boundary violators recover and avoid repeating their mistakes, Dr. Schenthal recreated himself and set out to teach others what he learned from his own violation.

With the support of others in the field, Dr. Schenthal founded Professional Boundaries, Inc. in 2001. Over the years, the company has grown to become the leader in remedial education for health care professionals and teachers facing disciplinary issues. In 2019, the company was renamed PBI Education. It now offers many different Continuing Medical Education/Continuing Education (CME/CE) courses, covering a wide range of topics. To date, PBI Education has helped safeguard thousands of medical professionals and the public they serve.

TABLE OF CONTENTS

About the Author

Acknowledgements

Preface

The Four Laws of Professional Boundaries

PART 1:
How Boundaries are Defined o How Boundaries are Enforced

How Boundaries are Enforced

The Forces

Warning Signs

Takeaways

PART 3:
Critical Moments in Your Career o Best Practices

Best Practices

Takeaways

PART 4:
Gauging Your Own Violation Potential o Putting the Formula to Work

Putting the Formula to Work

Takeaways

Afterword

ACKNOWLEDGEMENTS

I cannot hope to adequately thank all the people who have helped me over the years. I have learned from some of the best in the field, including Jennifer Schneider and Richard Irons, whose seminal book, *The Wounded Healer,* remains a classic. Marilyn Peterson's book, *At Personal Risk,* is so rich with insights and information that I have often recommended it to people in my classes. And Glen Gabbard's numerous books and articles have helped me immeasurably. I am grateful to these and other authors both for their published works and for their willingness to share their thoughts and ideas with me.

I am indebted, as well, to the talented professionals who have helped develop and lead PBI Education courses. Their devotion to the profession and concern for colleagues in pain is inspirational, and their experience and expertise have broadened my understanding of professional boundaries more than I can say. My special thanks to Jennifer Schneider and Catherine Caldicott for reading the manuscript of this book and helping to improve it.

Like all teachers, I continually learn from those I teach. Each new participant in our courses opens another window on the rapidly shifting challenges confronting today's health care professionals. And each new graduate reaffirms my faith in people's ability to confront those challenges and benefit from the experience.

Last but far from least, I have to thank Mark Schenthal, my brother and PBI Education's chief operating officer, for pushing me to finish the book I have been hoping to write

DR. STEPHEN SCHENTHAL

for longer than I care to remember.

PREFACE

When I ask physicians why they chose to become doctors, they give the same answer I gave when I first started practicing: I wanted to help, to heal. I was willing—no, eager—to spend my life easing pain and suffering.

My passion for medicine sustained me through all the years of training. When it was all over, I knew I would be a doctor like my father, someone people turned to for help, trusted completely, and admired without reservation. I saw how much it cost my dad—the long hours away from family and friends, the personal sacrifice—but I also saw how the profession sustained him. He went to bed each night exhausted, but he slept well, knowing he was a good doctor and a good person, selflessly dedicated to helping others in need. That's what I imagined for myself when I stood for the white coat ceremony after graduating medical school.

And then my license was revoked. Suddenly, instead of turning to me for help, people just turned away. Those who had admired me now scorned me. I felt worthless.

I remember asking myself how it was possible. I was a good person. All I ever wanted to do was help others. I was ethical and law-abiding. I mean, my first job out of college was as a cop! And yet I had betrayed my oath by causing harm, and I was now no longer allowed to practice medicine.

What I eventually came to realize is that the very qualities I had valued in myself, and that those around me valued so highly, were also liabilities.

- Without clearly established limits, my willingness to go above and beyond drove me to go too far.

- In my zeal to help, I denied my own limitations.
- I focused so intently on meeting my patients' needs, I lost my ability to say no.
- My self-sacrifice had become self-destructive.

I'm not suggesting that devotion and self-sacrifice aren't worthwhile. The danger comes from thinking they are sufficient. Properly harnessed, your passion for caring can make you a terrific doctor; unrestrained, it can tear you and your career apart.

Too often physicians wrap themselves up in a cocoon of goodness. Rather than consider the dark side of their virtues, their ability to do harm as well as good, they view their noble calling as a safe haven that offers a kind of professional invulnerability. "If I am selflessly devoted to helping my patients," they reason, "how can I possibly do anything to hurt them? I am nothing if not a good person so nothing I do can be bad."

This illusory sense of safety is a breeding ground for career-ending boundary violations.

I wrote this book to help you avoid such false security and achieve genuine safety. It distills much of what I have learned over more than two decades of working with physicians and other clinicians who have violated boundaries, often unknowingly and almost always with nothing but good intentions. And although this book was originally aimed at US physicians, its concepts and lessons are more broadly applicable to all clinicians. You will notice that much of the language in this book includes this broader audience in the US and Canada.

You are no doubt familiar with the term "professional boundaries," and probably have a vague sense of what it means. Perhaps in professional school you spent an hour or two in lectures on the subject. The first part of this book tells you everything they left out—how boundaries are defined, enforced, and what happens when they are violated.

In parts two and three, you'll learn about the forces that push good, ethical clinicians like you across professional boundaries, and about the basics of resisting those forces. In the final section, you'll learn how to gauge your own personal "violation potential" as it changes over the course of your career, and how to reduce it.

This same information has helped thousands who have attended PBI Education courses, almost always as a requirement of board (or the Canadian equivalent, a regulatory college) discipline. You now have a chance to learn what they learned without having to endure the months and often years of anguish they went through. Think of it as preventive medicine.

—Dr. Stephen Schenthal, CEO,
PBI Education

Note: *While loosely based on actual incidents, the events recounted in*

DR. STEPHEN SCHENTHAL

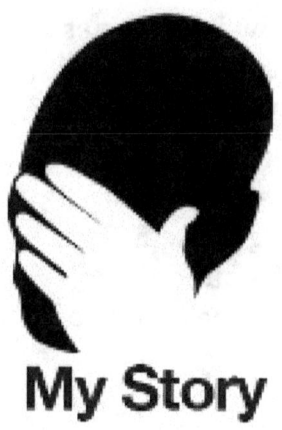

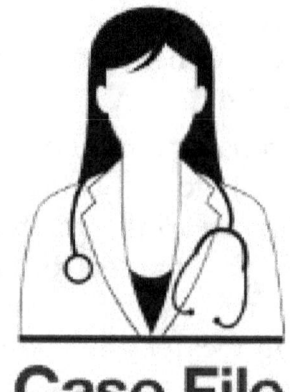

the Case File and My Story sections have been fictionalized to protect the identities of those involved.

THE FOUR LAWS OF PROFESSIONAL BOUNDARIES

#1 — Everyone Has A Violation Potential Which Is Constantly Changing.

You probably can't imagine being accused of a boundary violation, let alone committing one. Neither can most of the people who are sent by their board or regulatory college (collectively, a regulator) to our remedial three-day course on professional boundaries. Almost without exception, they start out defiant and enraged: "I don't belong here; this is all a big mistake... This is insane! I've been practicing for 20 years without a problem. My patients love me."

Then slowly, as they listen to each other's stories, these often highly successful professionals begin to see how even the best can get into serious trouble. Over the next three days, they learn things they never suspected—about boundaries they have crossed and personal issues they have kept hidden even from themselves. They start to see what went wrong and what might go wrong in the future. In the end, they come to realize the harsh reality expressed by the first law.

#2 — Perception Is 9/10 Of The Law.

If a patient thinks you have harmed them in some way, you're not likely to change their mind. And there is little chance you will persuade board members to believe you instead of your accuser. The board exists to protect your patients, not you or your license. If there is a possibility that you have abused your power and taken advantage of someone entrusted to your care, the board is going to side with the more vulnerable party.

Of course, board members are open to convincing, objective evidence. But it is far better to avoid an accusation in the first place, and to do that you need to embrace the essence of the second law: *If it looks bad, it is bad.*

#3 — Protect Yourself At All Times.

Without your license, your career is over. From that moment on, you are just a very smart unemployed person. Even if you only incur a six-month suspension, for those six months you will be without a source of income, simply another unemployed worker with non-transferable skills. Worse still, the loss of your license is likely to leave you without the sense of purpose your career provided. You can recover from this—most people do. But the recovery is slow and anguished.

The alternative is to realize that your career is fragile and needs to be continually protected.

This does not mean constantly looking over your shoulder or checking the rule book. Instead, as any good athlete knows, it means learning the rules well enough to be effective on the field without committing any penalties.

You're no help to anyone if you're no longer in the game.

#4 — The Board (Or College) Decides What's Right, Not You.

If you are accused of a boundary violation, your case will not be decided in the civil or criminal courts of law you learned about in school. When you appear before your regulatory board or agency, you enter the domain of administrative law. Here, the same agency that makes the rules enforces them. You have the right to an attorney, but unless you reach a settlement with the board, your case will be heard either by board members themselves or by an administrative law judge. Even the judge's ruling is subject to board approval. In Canada, the procedure is similar. An administrative decision-maker, such as a tribunal of a regulatory college, will hear your case. The tribunal has the power to enforce its decision itself, although a court could provide a judicial review, but only on procedural matters.

So no matter how convinced you are that your accuser has failed to prove the charges, that the preponderance of evidence is in your favor, or that any fair jury of your peers would find you not guilty, it is the board or college that will decide your fate. There are limited rights of appeal, but they are rarely successful.

Physicians disciplined by their regulators almost always arrive at our remedial courses convinced that they have been treated unfairly. Over the years, we have learned to

let them vent their anger and frustration. Only then are they prepared to accept the validity of the fourth law: *Ultimately, the board or college decides what's right, not you.*

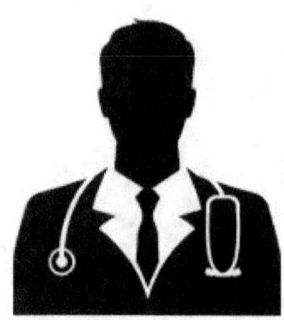

Case File

Dr. Gregory had been in practice for more than 20 years. Known as a devoted and caring physician, he was adored by his patients and proud of his long, unblemished career. When his wife was badly injured in a car accident, he managed to tend to her needs without shortchanging his patients. It was exhausting but the gratitude and admiration he earned made it all worthwhile.

Rather than let tickets to a charity ball go unused, Dr. Gregory offered them to patients he thought might enjoy the occasion. It was against office policy to exchange gifts with patients, but he saw no harm in being generous. The first few thanked him but were unable to take advantage of the offer. Monica, however, was delighted and eagerly accepted.

When she asked what she should wear, Dr. Gregory took the opportunity to compliment her good taste and told her he was sure she would look beautiful in whatever she wore. But when Monica asked who should drive, Dr. Gregory realized there had been a misunderstanding. He quickly explained that the tickets were a gift, not an invitation to share an evening out. Monica blushed in embarrassment, apologized and left quickly. A few days later she called to cancel an appointment and before long, Dr. Gregory learned Monica had shifted to another practice. He called to apologize, but Monica never returned his calls.

Then one day, he received a letter from his board. Monica had filed a complaint, saying Dr. Gregory had been flirting with her and offered her a gift. Appearing before the board, he denied ever flirting and explained both his *selfless efforts to continue working despite his wife's accident and his good intentions in offering the tickets.*

After listening to his side of the story, the board told the physician he had used poor judgment in offering the tickets to patients, and reminded him that he was responsible for managing his professional relationship with Monica. The board also cautioned him about over-extending himself. Exhaustion, they said, might well have contributed to Dr. Gregory's violation, but he was responsible for that too. By trying to take care of everyone, both his wife and his patients, Dr. Gregory had overextended himself. In the future, for the good of his patients, he should recognize his limitations and adjust his activities accordingly.

Dr. Gregory's license was suspended for six months.

The Four Laws of Professional Boundaries

Everyone has a violation potential which is constantly changing.

Perception is 9/10 of the law.

Protect yourself at all times.

The board (or college) decides what's right, not you.

PART 1:
Understanding Professional Boundaries

How Boundaries Are Defined o How Boundaries Are Enforced

It may not always feel like it, but as a clinician, you have enormous power over your patients. You can ask them questions no one else would dare ask, and they answer, often without hesitation. Patients tell you things about themselves they haven't even revealed to their families. They disrobe when you ask them to; let you poke and prod them as you see fit; inject them with foreign substances and draw their blood. And when you tell them what's wrong with them, and what they should do to get better, they generally respect your judgment and follow your advice. They put their health, sometimes even their lives, in your hands.

To ensure that you are worthy of this trust, your jurisdiction —a state, province, or territory—holds you to the highest legal standard of care: fiduciary responsibility. At the most basic level, that means always putting your patient's interests ahead of your own. The word "fiduciary" comes from the Latin word for "trust," and describes a relationship that cannot exist without it. Your patients may not know about the fiduciary rule, but they believe they can trust you to always do what's best for them because you are a licensed clinician. Maintaining that trust is your primary professional obligation and a condition of your licensure.

Professional boundaries define the limits of professionalism. As you're about to learn, some of these limits are explicitly codified; others are more subjective. But all professional boundaries are expressions of your fiduciary obligation to your patients. They restrict your words and actions to ensure that you are always putting your patient's needs first, and never acting out of self-interest.

You inflict harm when you violate professional boundaries. All this talk of fiduciary obligation and professionalism risks dehumanizing the real pain boundary violations cause patients. Sexual boundary violations are the ones most often covered by the media and most analyzed by researchers. Numerous studies have shown that patients who have sex with their doctor, whether or not they consider it consensual, suffer in numerous ways.

> *"Victims fluctuate between rage and despair but are often unable to talk about the source of their rage. Suicidal risk increases and cognitive deficits such as inattention, intrusive thoughts, flashbacks, and nightmares are common. Simple daily tasks may seem impossible to perform. A variety of diagnoses afflict these victims, including posttraumatic stress disorder, major depression, anxiety states and panic disorder, eating disorders, and drug and alcohol abuse. Also, personality disorders which had lain dormant may become aggravated."*[1]

If the patient has suffered abuse before, either as a child or an adult—by no means uncommon—the trauma is all the more severe.

Despite the media's obsession, the vast majority of violations have nothing to do with sexual activity. That doesn't make them any less harmful. Among the most serious consequences of all violations, sexual or not, is the loss of trust. Patients may become so distrustful of physicians or other clinicians that they stop seeking out health care when they need it. At the very least, they lose the care of a clinician they have trusted and who is often the person most knowledgeable about their medical needs.

This sense of betrayal is compounded by the trust and openness patients bring to the relationship—the same trust and openness the fiduciary obligation was created to defend—and from the idealization that commonly accompanies such trust. One physician assistant who eventually realized what he had done, explained it like this:

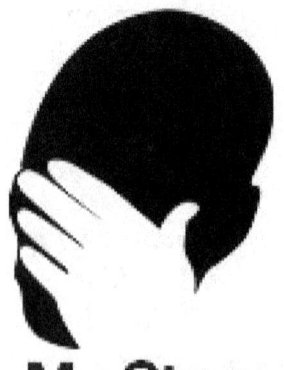

"Patients come with a need to have someone they consider safe, smart, perfect. It does not that it's not based on reality or that you can't avoid disappointing them. Patients are bound to be disappointed by me at times, as they come to see my human failings. But those bite-sized pieces of disillusionment are very different from the massive disappointment and disillusionment of a betrayal. It took me a long time to understand the devastation I caused by betraying that idealization and even longer to forgive myself."

How Boundaries Are Defined

Think of professional boundaries as an all-encompassing sphere established to protect both you and those who put their trust in you. The sphere's limits are defined by external forces: federal and state or provincial laws, hospital by-laws, professional codes of ethics, as well as social and cultural norms. Together, these regulations and constraints create the Boundary Sphere, which defines the scope of professional behavior your patients have a right to expect of you.

As long as you remain within this Boundary Sphere, your internal desire to help is a positive force, driving you to do all you can for your patients. But the moment your personal needs begin to take precedence, the moment you begin to consider your own interests when making decisions about a patient, you are at risk of piercing the sphere, of violating professional boundaries.

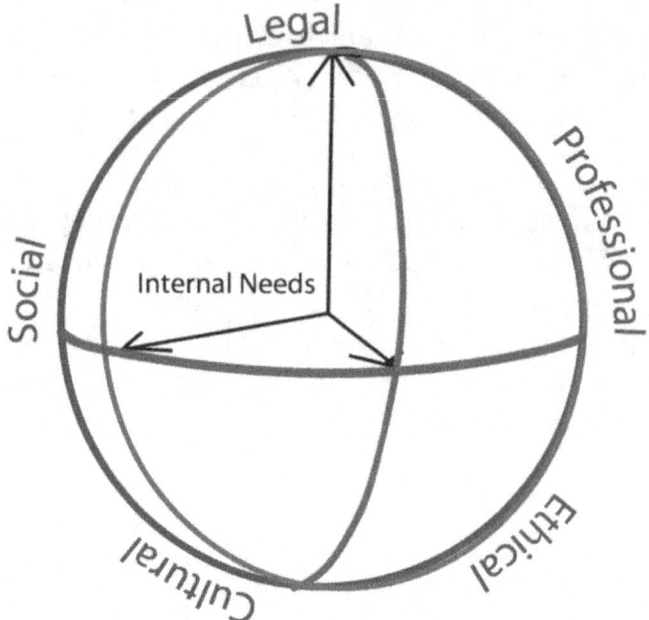

The Boundary Sphere

You are not the best judge of your own motivations. In the heat of the moment, you may honestly believe you need to push through a boundary for the good of your patient. Many who have lost their license felt the same way. The reality is that, like all human beings, your own needs can blind you to your true motivation. Consider the following case:

THE PHYSICIAN'S GUIDE TO PROFESSIONAL BOUNDARIES

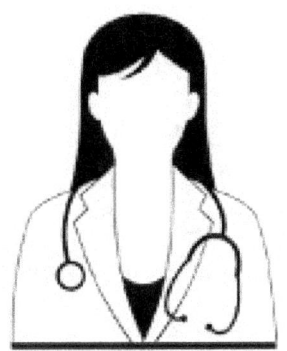

Case File

Dr. Jones had been a hospitalist for several years. She prided herself on her professionalism and was well liked both by patients and by their personal physicians. When patients were discharged, she wished them well and moved on.

In Joe's case though, Dr. Jones felt a special bond. Joe was an elderly patient with early dementia and Dr. Jones was concerned that he might not get the home care he needed after his stay in the hospital. She had spoken to Joe's daughter who welcomed her concern and invited her to stop by to see how her father was doing.

Her first visit went well, but when Dr. Jones realized Joe had forgotten to fill a recent prescription, she ran over to the pharmacy to pick it up for him. The next day, she stopped by again to check on him. The home visits soon became a regular part of the doctor's routine. On one occasion, when Joe complained of untreated pain, Dr. Jones prescribed medication without consulting the family or family doctor. Had she discussed his concerns with either of them, she would have learned that they were working to wean Joe off pain meds, suspecting that his dependence on them was worsening his dementia.

When Joe's regular doctor heard about the unauthorized prescription, he complained both to Dr. Jones and to the hospital where she worked. The hospital suspended Dr. Jones for treating a patient after discharge, the family sued, and the medical liability insurance carrier refused to cover the cost of the settlement because Dr. Jones was practicing outside the hospital.

Throughout all this, Dr. Jones was confident she was work-

> ing in Joe's best interest, but after discussing the situation with a counselor, she realized that she had been motivated by her own needs. Her elderly father had died recently and she blamed herself for not taking better care of him. Dr. Jones honestly thought she had moved past the grief and guilt, but now saw that it had been pushing her to go beyond the boundaries of her job to care for Joe.

Professional boundaries are like buoys warning ships of hidden hazards. No matter how convinced we are of our course at any given moment, it is never wise to ignore the buoys.

Some Professional Boundaries Are Explicitly Defined In Writing

These rules and regulations tell you what is not allowed: no sexual contact with patients, no breach of confidentiality, no charging for unnecessary work. Such prohibitions "explicitly define the standards that are intended to safeguard the client's trust by restricting the professional's power," says Marilyn Peterson, author of *At Personal Risk*.

> "For example, rules about confidentiality attempt to guard the client's privacy by restricting the professional's freedom of disclosure. Rules about conflicts of interest tend to guard the primacy of the client's need by restricting the professional's self-interest."[2]

Each state in the U.S. has its own Professional Practice Act, which regulates the conduct of health professionals (as well as defining the requirements for licensure and the board's powers). Examples would be a state's medical practice act, dental practice act, nursing practice act, etc. Similarly, each Canadian province and territory has its own Regulated Health Professions Act (RHPA) that gives regulatory colleges the power and duty to oversee the practice of each of the health professions. These laws vary slightly from jurisdiction to jurisdiction, but all clearly establish the limits of professional conduct. According to the Federation of State Medical Boards, examples of unprofessional conduct include the following:

- Alcohol and substance abuse
- Sexual misconduct
- Neglect of a patient
- Failing to meet the accepted standard of care in a state
- Prescribing drugs in excess or without a legitimate reason
- Dishonesty during the license application process
- Conviction of a felony
- Fraud
- Delegating the practice of medicine to an unlicensed individual
- Inadequate record keeping
- Failing to meet continuing medical education requirements

If you are like most clinicians, you haven't read your state's Professional Practice Act or province's RHPA that pertains to your health profession—at least not recently, and possibly not ever. After all, you've devoted years of your life to becoming an independent clinician, spending endless hours in lecture halls and laboratories, passing stringent exams, and caring for patients under the watchful eyes of experienced supervisors. Of course, you believe you know what's required of you and what's prohibited. Between your years of training and your innate sense of right and wrong, you are confident of your professionalism.

But consider something as basic as medical records. Can you honestly answer the following questions with complete confidence?

- Do you know how long you are required to keep patients' medical records? Does your answer vary depending on the type of insurance involved?

- Are your patient notes "complete" as currently defined by board or college rules?

- Do you document every time a patient calls with a quick question?

- What kind of documentation is required for a routine prescription refill? What if the medication is an opioid?

If you haven't recently checked your jurisdiction's rules, there's a good chance at least one of your answers to these questions is wrong and that your mistake could result in civil penalties and/or disciplinary action.

So don't make the common mistake of thinking you don't need to know the rules, or don't have the time to learn them. You wouldn't think of not keeping up with the latest research in your field. Not keeping up with your state's Medical Practice Act or province's RHPA—which the legislature can change at any time—is just as reckless. You'll find it on your board's or regulatory college's website (see **Resources** at the end of this section). Don't be intimidated by the length. The entries are short and easily scanned.

You are also subject to relevant civil and criminal laws. There are three types of law in the United States. While administrative law governs the board and your license, civil law governs disputes between individuals, including malpractice suits and breaches of contract. Financial compensation is the most common remedy when there is a violation of civil law. Criminal law protects society from those who would harm others. Cases are prosecuted by the government and penalties include both fines and imprisonment. The legal system in Canada is a bit different, and is divided into public and private (or civil) law. Public law includes criminal, constitutional, and administrative. Administrative law addresses activities of regulatory colleges, as noted above under Law #4.

Federal law. If prosecutors believe you have violated any of the federal laws governing your practice, you will end up in criminal court where you will face hefty fines, additional charges based on the amounts involved, and potential imprisonment. In addition, criminal charges and/or conviction virtually guarantee board or regulator action.

There are three major areas of federal law governing health care professionals. Here's a brief high-level overview of a sometimes daunting landscape.

- **HIPAA (Health Insurance Portability and Accountability Act) in the US.** As the name suggests, HIPAA is designed to safeguard patients' privacy and their right to access their own medical records. Since it was first enacted in 1996, the law has been changed numerous times. Among other things, recent revisions have addressed changes in technology. To be in compliance with HIPAA rules, your office must conduct annual HIPAA audits; correct any gaps the audit identifies; establish policies and procedures safeguarding protected health information (and ensure that patients are aware of them and employees are trained to follow them); manage vendor access to patient information; report incidents; and document actions taken to remain in compliance.

  Canada's federal law, PIPEDA (Personal Information Protection and Electronic Documents Act) is in some

ways comparable to HIPAA. However, unlike HIPAA, PIPEDA governs all personal data, not just health related information. PIPEDA does not apply in all provinces; a province may choose to set its own rules and regulations regarding data privacy, as long as they are substantially similar to PIPEDA. You should be familiar with the data protection standards that apply in your province, whether they are PIPEDA or something else.

Controlled Substances Act in the US; Controlled Drugs and Substances Act in Canada. To prescribe any of the drugs cataloged in the law (and the list is subject to change), you must be fully licensed to handle controlled substances by the state(s) or province(s) in which you practice. Even then, you are only allowed to prescribe a controlled substance for "a legitimate medical purpose" within "the usual course of professional practice."[3] Neither of these requirements is clearly defined and both are open to interpretation. It is your responsibility to stay abreast of any changes in the law and understand how it is enforced in your area. It is also up to you to recognize warning signs that indicate a patient may be abusing a prescription and take appropriate action (see **10 Warning Signs of Patient Drug Abuse**).

10 Warning Signs of Patient Drug Abuse[4]

If The Patient...

1. Declines a physical exam and diagnostic tests and won't give the clinician permission to obtain past records
2. Travels an exceptionally long distance or out

of state or province for the visit and doesn't explain why
3. Repeatedly seeks medications from non-coordinated sites such as emergency rooms, urgent care centers, or walk-in clinics
4. Obtains prescriptions from multiple providers without the prescribers' knowledge (this information is available through Prescription Drug Monitoring Programs)
5. Repeatedly resists changes in the treatment plan despite evidence of adverse physical or psychological effects from the drug
6. Repeatedly claims to have lost their prescription or medication
7. Refuses to try nonpharmacologic therapies and won't explain why
8. Attempts to alter, forge, or rewrite prescriptions
9. Diverts or sells medication or borrows drugs from others
10. Requests prescriptions written in the names of other people for whom the physician is not the designated caregiver.

Caveat: There is no substitute for getting to know your patient. A warning sign does not automatically indicate a problem. There may well be an innocent explanation. The only way to find out is to talk to your patient.

Medicare/Medicaid Fraud and Abuse Laws. Key statutes include:

- False Claims Act makes it illegal to submit claims for payment to Medicare or Medicaid that you know or should know are false or fraudulent. In Canada, Medicare is the name of the publicly funded health care system. Submission of false or fraudulent claims are illegal and could lead to the suspension or revocation of a clinician's certificate of registration, in addition to large fines.

- Physician Self-Referral Law (Stark Law) in the US prohibits you from referring Medicare or Medicaid patients to any place where you have a financial relationship. Canada does not have a Stark Law equivalent. Self-referral is generally considered professional misconduct by regulators.

- Anti-Kickback Statute explicitly rules out taking money or gifts from a drug or device company or a durable medical equipment (DME) supplier. Similar to above, clinicians accepting kickbacks are considered to be committing professional misconduct.

Exclusion Authorities: In the US, if either service excludes you from its list of approved providers, you may not bill Medicare or Medicaid either directly or indirectly.

A Federal System Without The Federal Government

Inter-state enforcement of discipline in the US: To prevent US physicians from escaping disciplinary actions by simply moving to another state, the Federation of State Medical Boards (FSMB) created the Physician Data Center, which the Federation describes as, "A comprehensive data repository that contains information about the nearly one million actively licensed physicians in the United States, as well as board disciplinary actions dating back to the early 1960s."[5] Currently the Federation of Medical Regulatory Authorities in Canada does not maintain a similar repository.

Medical boards use this database to vet new applicants for licensure and, "The Data Center's Disciplinary Alert Service proactively alerts all states in which a disciplined physician is licensed within 24-48 hours after a disciplinary action taken by one of those states has been reported." It's up to each state to decide how to respond—whether to mirror the discipline, for instance, or perhaps take stronger measures.

Inter-state or inter-province licensing for telemedicine: Telemedicine makes it possible for patients to be "seen" by a clinician even if there isn't one available to them locally. Unfortunately, it's not uncommon for the patient and clinician to be on opposite sides of a state or province line, which means the clinician has to be licensed in both states in the US, and potentially both provinces in Canada. Under current US law, a clinician has to go through the often lengthy licensing process state by state. Canadian physicians should check with the regulator in their province and in the province of the patient to ensure they comply with the current standards of practice in both jurisdictions.

In 2013 FSMB organized a team of state medical board representatives and experts from the Council of State Governments (CSG) to draft an Interstate Medical Licensure Compact — a new expedited licensing option for qualified physicians seeking to practice in multiple states. As of July 2020, 29 states and the District of Columbia and Guam have signed onto the Compact. Currently, there is no interprovincial medical licensure compact in Canada. Nurses in the US also have an interstate licensure compact in which 33 states currently participate.

Dr. Parsons was proud of the practice he had built up over the years. He saw patients in two different offices and had highly qualified physician assistants seeing patients in both locations. As his patient list grew, he realized he needed help with the paperwork and hired a well-regarded vendor in the area. Before long, his paperwork had been reduced to a quick review of monthly summaries provided

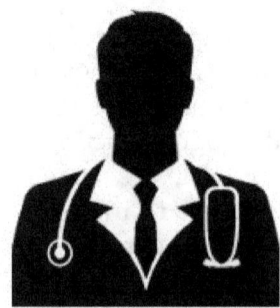

Case File

by the billing company.

It was not until his insurance company audited his practice that Dr. Parsons found out all of the practitioners at both offices had been billing under his name, which made it look like he was billing for services he could not possibly have provided. Following the audit, the FBI demanded copies of billing sheets and patient charts. In short order, Dr. Parsons was indicted by a grand jury on multiple counts of medical and wire fraud.

He lost the case in court and the judge gave him the shortest prison term he could under federal sentencing guidelines—a year and a day. Had Dr. Parsons been convicted on all counts, he could have received more than 20 years.

He lost the case in court and the judge gave him the shortest prison term he could under federal sentencing guidelines—a year and a day. Had Dr. Parsons been convicted on all counts, he could have received more than 20 years.

The board revoked his license to practice and the state took away his license to prescribe controlled substances. After serving his term and completing extensive remedial education, Dr. Parsons earned back both licenses. But all health insurance companies excluded him from their lists of approved providers, which severely limited the patients willing to see him.

Other Boundaries Are Less Rigidly Defined

The boundaries that are specifically defined in law, such as fraud and conflicts of interest, are generally classified as *administrative boundaries*. The term *professional boundaries* is more often reserved for situations involving human relationships, like the one between a patient and a clinician. Given the practical impossibility of defining rules for every possible situation that might arise in clinician-patient relationships, virtually all state and provincial Professional Practice Acts (e.g., Medical Practice Act, Dental Practice Act, Nursing Act, Physiotherapy Act, etc.) include a catch-all category that allows regulators to make case-by-case decisions, whether or not the behavior they object to is explicitly forbidden in writing.

Dual Relationships. Anything that potentially compromises your fiduciary obligation is considered problematic by your regulator. The most common issue is a non-medical or non-clinical relationship between you and your patient. Whether it is romantic, personal, social, or business-related, any "dual relationship" jeopardizes your clinical objectivity and single-minded focus on what's best for your patient's health. It doesn't matter how innocent the non-medical relationship may seem, or how diligently you try to prevent it from affecting your professional judgment. Any relationship you have with a patient other than as their healthcare provider weakens the primacy of the clinician-patient relationship.

It happens every day: someone on staff stops you in the hall and says they have a sinus infection or that their reflux is acting up. They ask you for a prescription or perhaps some samples off the shelf in the office. You may ask a couple of quick questions, but you're in a hurry, as are they, so you do as they ask and move on—unaware of the risks you've taken.

If a patient came to you with the same complaint, saying they had sinusitis or reflux, you would take a history, examine them, perhaps do a diagnostic maneuver or order labs or studies, offer clinical advice, answer any questions, address any concerns, arrange for appropriate follow-up and write everything down in their chart. Chances are you did none of these things when you "helped out" your colleague in the hallway. So if anything goes amiss—a bad reaction to the medication, or complications from an undiagnosed condition—you are in deep trouble. Depending on the seriousness of the situation, you could face criminal charges, a malpractice suit, and professional sanction or discipline up to and including the loss of your license.

From the board's or college's perspective, the primary problem is not simply the potential harm you may have caused this "patient" or your failure to adhere to what the lawyers call "standard of care." The board's or college's fundamental concern is the "dual relationship" (personal and professional) you now have with your colleague/patient.

Dual relationships are not always easy to avoid. It's not uncommon, for instance, for clinicians and patients to know each other outside the office, especially in small communities. And in most cases, there's no problem as long as the clinician and patient both understand the differences between their personal and professional relationships and respect the boundaries between the two realms—although it's up to the clinician to remain vigilant and refer the patient to another provider if boundary issues emerge. The problem arises when the non-clinical relationship threatens to compromise the clinician- patient relationship.

> *Andrea Frank, a nurse practitioner, was herself a victim, having recently ended an abusive relationship. In addition to the emotional turmoil involved, she was also increasingly anxious about her personal finances. She was still paying off considerable student debt and now was also incurring hefty bills from the lawyer and therapist working with her.*
>
> *When Sam, a well-to-do, long-time patient, noticed a wor-*

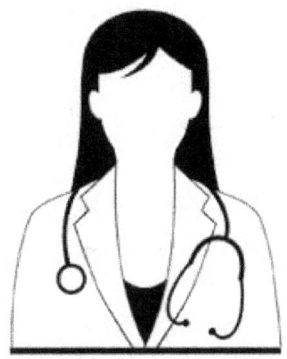

Case File

ried look on Andrea's face, he asked if something was wrong. She briefly mentioned her predicament, and Sam offered her a personal interest-free loan. After a good deal of coaxing, she accepted it. Andrea soon regained control of her finances and paid back the loan in full.

Sam was pleased to have helped. His wife was not. She had seen Sam lend money casually many times before, often with bad results. She was angry at her husband but also felt he had been exploited by Ms. Frank. She complained to the nursing board.

In their disciplinary order, the board expressed concern about the dual relationship Ms. Frank had allowed to develop. They noted that she had reversed roles with her patient by accepting his help for her problem, and exacerbated a problem he himself was struggling with. By entering into a non-medical business relationship with Sam, she had both jeopardized her own professional objectivity and interfered with his marital relationship.

Ms. Frank's license was suspended for two years.

Treating colleagues and friends. The hallway encounter is just one example of the complications that can arise from dual relationships. Consider another workplace scenario. A colleague makes an appointment and comes to see you as a patient. Even assuming you treat them as you would any other patient, you are still exposing yourself and your patient to considerable risks.

"When I see a friend or colleague as a patient, I'm both doctor and friend (or colleague), and the dual role may lead me to do too much or too little," says Mark A. Graber, MD, professor of emergency and family medicine at the University of Iowa Carver College of Medicine.

> "On the one hand, I may pursue investigations to the nth degree to avoid an error in diagnosis or treatment; I'm too invested in the outcome of this patient. My attitude may cause me to order unnecessary tests, with the patient bearing the attendant risk. For example, I may order a stress test on a low-risk colleague or friend—just to be sure. The result is a false positive, which leads to an invasive cardiac catheterization.
>
> "On the other hand, I may have so great an emotional connection with the patient that I do too little. I may avoid potentially painful procedures that I would do if I were guided by more objective clinical judgment. I may perform a lumbar puncture for an "ordinary" patient with a headache and fever without a second thought but may be loath to do one on a friend. Friendship can cloud our judgment."[6]

Treating family members. Rather than bringing a sick spouse or injured child to the family doctor, clinicians often handle the situation themselves, especially if the family member is in pain or the family doctor's office is closed. Why make someone you love wait for relief when you can instantly provide first-rate compassionate care free of charge?

Although the practice is common, virtually all professional organizations—including the American College of Physicians, the American Academy of Pediatrics and the American and Canadian Medical Associations (AMA and CMA)—warn physicians away from treating family members. The AMA's Code of Ethics has discouraged the practice since it was first drafted in 1847.

The prohibition is not absolute. According to the AMA's

Code of Medical Ethics (Opinion 8.19), "Physicians should not hesitate to treat themselves or family members until another physician becomes available. In addition, while physicians should not serve as a primary or regular care provider for immediate family members, there are situations in which routine care is acceptable for short-term, minor problems."[7] When it comes to pain management, however, the AMA cautions physicians not to prescribe controlled substances for family members except in extreme emergencies.

Among the many reasons to avoid treating family members, the Texas Medical Association includes the following:

- Professional objectivity may be compromised.

- Physicians' personal feelings may unduly influence their professional medical judgment, thereby interfering with the care being delivered.

- Physicians may fail to probe sensitive areas when taking the medical history or may fail to perform intimate parts of the physical examination.

- Patients may feel uncomfortable disclosing sensitive information or undergoing an intimate examination when the physician is an immediate family member.

- Physicians may be inclined to treat problems that are beyond their expertise or training.

- Family members may be reluctant to state their preference for another physician or decline a recommendation for fear of offending the family member/physician.

- Physicians may feel obligated to provide care to immediate family members even if they feel uncomfortable providing care.

Behind each of these reasons stretch numerous examples of family treatment gone wrong.

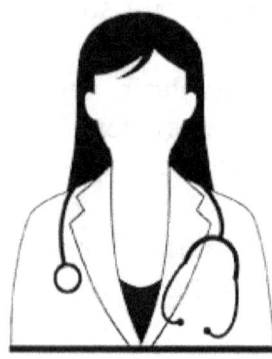

Case File

Dr. Smith was an ob-gyn, but when her son came down with a fever and abdominal pain one weekend, it seemed crazy to bring him to some urgent-care clinic at a mall. She knew what the problem was, so she wrote a prescription and spent the day with him. By evening, he was getting worse and she ended up taking him to the ER. Dr. Smith had misdiagnosed her son. Realizing she had put him at risk, she self-reported to her board. At the hearing, she had to admit she had not taken a history, consulted her son's chart or recorded what she had done. She was also "out of scope." Her license was suspended for six months.

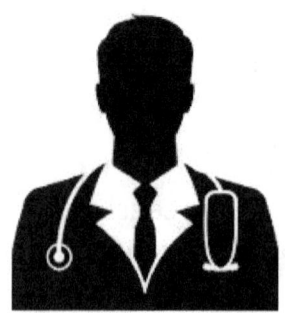

Case File

When he and his family moved to an area without local psychiatric help, it seemed reasonable to Dr. Benjamin, a dental surgeon, that he provide "bridge care" for his wife. She was taking antidepressants to help with anxiety and OCD, and when she ran out, Dr. Benjamin wrote her a new prescription. Although he explained the situation to the pharmacist, he didn't put anything in her chart. The pharmacist expressed discomfort about filling the prescription, but let it slide.

A few weeks later, when his wife's psychiatric symptoms worsened, Dr. Benjamin upped her antidepressant until she could get an appointment with a licensed psychiatrist. This time the pharmacist reported him to the board (or regulatory college) for prescribing outside his scope of practice. In the *disciplinary order suspending his license for two years, the regulator stated, "If this is an example of your clinical judgment, we have to question your judgment with all your patients."*

Not all dual relationships end badly. Indeed, most pass unnoticed. But the potential for harm, both to the clinician and the patient, is real, which is why the American College of Physicians' Ethics Manual offers this advice: "If a physician does treat a close friend, family member, or employee out of necessity, the patient should be transferred to another physician as soon as it is practical... Otherwise, requests for care on the part of employees, family members, or friends should be resolved by assisting them in obtaining appropriate care."[8]

Self-treatment is also frowned upon as a kind of internal dual relationship. You cannot hope to be objective in caring for yourself. The risks of unconsciously steering clear of serious issues or pursuing minor ones to unprofessional lengths are equally compelling. A lawyer who defends them self is said to have a fool for a client. Clinicians who treat themselves suffer doubly, both as the patient (who gets inadequate care) and as the clinician (who fails to live up to professional standards).

Personal involvement with patients. In all of the cases just covered, the non-clinical relationship—with colleagues, friends, and family—came first. But of course, dual relationships can also arise in the course of treating regular patients. Clinicians and patients are human beings with blind spots, needs and personal problems. Given the degree of physical contact and emotional content involved in many clinician-patient relationships, it's not surprising that strong feelings can develop.

It was a routine follow-up after treatment for a sinus

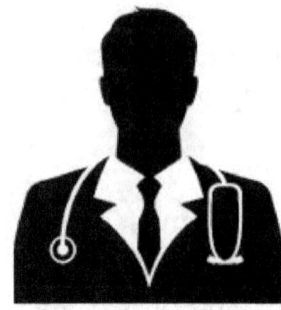

Case File

infection, but judging from the patient's appearance, the antibiotics had not worked. Beth's eyes were red and swollen and she was congested. It did not take long for George Spencer, a physician assistant, to realize the problem was emotional, not medical.

Beth told him her father had died unexpectedly and she was having trouble accepting the loss. As she stood to leave, Beth started sobbing.

George gave her a tissue and tried to offer words of comfort, but she continued crying. After a few minutes, he placed his hand on her shoulder. She collapsed into him and before he knew it, he was hugging her. Eventually, Beth regained her composure, apologized and left the office.

For days afterward, George found himself thinking of that hug. When his wife asked why he seemed so preoccupied, he told her it was a troubling case and tried to brush the whole thing off. But the more he thought about it, the more sure he was that the hug meant something more to Beth, too.

Eager to see her again, George called Beth, ostensibly to see how she was doing. She was still very distraught and he invited her to come in to discuss grief counseling options. When she sat down next to him in the office, Beth put her hand on his knee as she thanked him for his kindness.

As the appointment was drawing to a close, George felt the time was right and asked Beth if she would like to join him for a drink sometime. Beth flushed with embarrassment, stammered a hasty apology for having given him the wrong idea and rushed out. George tried to apologize, but Beth let his calls go to voicemail.

When she called a few days later asking for a referral to a new medical practice, the receptionist asked why and Beth explained what had happened. Word got back to one of George's partners in the practice, who reported George to the board. George had his license suspended for a year and was required to attend an ethics course and seek counseling before returning to work.

The situation is no less harmful when both patient and clinician say they feel the same way about one another. What too many clinicians forget—if they ever knew—is that, according to the AMA and virtually all state medical boards and regulatory colleges, there is no such thing as a consensual sexual or romantic relationship between a clinician and a patient. According to a 2013 article in the *New York Law Journal*, "Studies have proven that the physician's tremendous power over the patient, coupled with the patient's emotional and/or psychological vulnerability, deprives the patient of the ability to give true or valid consent to a sexual relationship with her physician." The article goes on to cite a 1991 AMA report, which notes, "'The lack of reliable or true consent on the part of the patient...has led researchers to compare physician-patient sexual contact with other sexually exploitative situations such as sexual assault and incest.'"[9]

Dr. Sandra Malone, an ob-gyn, had been friends with Gwen, a long-time patient, for several years. They had discussed the potential conflicts between their personal and professional relationships and both agreed they were comfortable with the arrangement.

Privately, the friends frequently discussed their per-

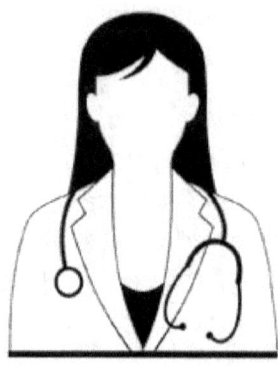

Case File

sonal lives. Gwen was openly gay and married. But when Dr. Malone complained about her husband's constant travel, Gwen confided that her own spouse spent so much time at the office, she was hardly ever home. Over time, as the two friends discussed their problems, they grew closer. Eventually, they confessed their feelings for each other and began to see each other romantically.

When their relationship became intimate, both agreed to tell their spouses. Gwen and her spouse quickly agreed to separate. Dr. Malone's husband, however, became enraged and, among other things, threatened to report her to the medical board. Panicked, she told Gwen they would have to slow things down. Hurt and angry, Gwen filed a complaint, and the board revoked Dr. Malone's license.

How Boundaries Are Enforced

The board's or college's duty is to protect the public, not you. State health professional boards and Canadian regulatory colleges were created to protect the public—initially from the numerous charlatans and hacks who chose to call themselves doctors or healers of other sorts. At first, that meant licensing clinicians so people would know who the honest practitioners were. Later, the boards focused on raising the standards of the professions by requiring clinicians to pass exams. More recently, the focus has shifted to weeding out clinicians who violate professional standards after obtaining a license. Today, responding to complaints and taking disciplinary action (if warranted) is considered a significant part of boards' mandates.

You may believe that your license gives you the right to practice. It doesn't. Legally, rights are guaranteed by the state and can be curtailed only by due process of law. The same is not true of your professional license. The state or province/territory defines your license to practice as a privilege, not a right, and the state board or regulatory college that granted your license can revoke it whenever it determines that doing so is prudent. The moment you give the board or college any reason to suspect you lack the necessary professionalism to safely serve your patients, you put your license at risk.

Boards and colleges are under increasing pressure to aggressively weed out and discipline violators. In fact, one nationwide consumer group in the U.S., Public Citizen, rates medical boards according to how many physicians they seriously discipline each year, and the press often alerts the public to boards that reporters believe are being too lenient.

Virtually anyone can file a complaint with a licensing board or regulatory college—patients, peers, staff, hospitals, clinics, pharmacists, and/or insurance companies. Every complaint is carefully considered on a regular basis. Board members are far less concerned with what a patient may have done to provoke a violation or what might be motivating their complaint. They hold you, the clinician, responsible for managing your relationship with your patients, regardless of their behavior or motivations. As mentioned earlier, if it comes down to your word against your patient's, the board is far more likely to side with the more vulnerable party. If the accusation is serious enough, and board members have reason to believe you may pose an imminent threat to the public, they will immediately suspend your license until an investigation has been completed and a hearing can be held.

If the board or college decides to investigate the complaint, its investigators pursue many of the same avenues that police do when investigating a criminal complaint, and with much the same authority. They conduct interviews, gather physical evidence, including medical and pharmacy records if necessary, and work together with federal, state or provincial, and local law enforcement when appropriate. Some regulators employ counterfeit patients to test clinicians' compliance, especially when they suspect sexual violations or drug abuse. And when boards or colleges feel the situation warrants force, they may even call in the police, including armed SWAT teams, to shut down suspect practices.

In the US, if the board decides to file charges, the clinician can request a settlement conference, during which the clinician and their attorney meet with the representatives of the board to discuss options. If an agreement is reached, the board will issue an order, commonly called a consent decree, agreement or an agreed order in the US.

In Canada, if the investigation findings suggest professional misconduct or incompetence (as defined in the RHPA), a disciplinary hearing will be held. (If the licensee disagrees with the decision of the complaints committee, they can request a review, which may be undertaken by a member of the College administration, such as the Registrar.) The College Disciplinary Committee or Hearing Tribunal will make a decision on the case. If both the College and the member (licensee) agree on an Agreed Statement of Facts, a Joint Submission on Sanction (or Penalty) will constitute the orders imposed on the licensee. For lesser offenses that do not rise to the level of needing formal discipline, the regulatory College may draw up a Memorandum of Understanding or an Undertaking based on the investigation findings alone, which the member can sign as a settlement of the matter.

The reason so many clinicians prefer to take the settlement route is that it's quicker, easier, and less expensive. One disadvantage of settlement agreements is that they preclude the possibility of an appeal, since both parties agreed to the judgment ahead of time. (In the US, in the case of a hearing, the clinician can appeal the board's decision in civil court, although board decisions are rarely reversed. Canadian licensees can appeal the decisions of a college discipline committee, too, in an administrative court. However, if their legal representation was from the Canadian Medical Protective Association (CMPA), the CMPA normally only assists in an appeal if there was an issue in how disciplinary procedure was followed. As in the US, college decisions are rarely reversed in the appeals process.) There are other potential downsides to a settlement, as well. These vary from case to case, but can include the creation of a public record, loss of insurance contracts, loss of specialty board certification and increased malpractice rates.

In the US, if an agreement is not reached or the clinician chooses to contest the charges, a formal hearing, known as an administrative tribunal or hearing, is held. Such hearings are similar to a civil trial, but there are important differences. Witnesses are questioned by both sides and evidence is presented, for example, but there is no presumption of innocence and the burden of proof is a preponderance of the evidence, meaning 51%. An administrative law judge presides over the proceedings but is not the final decision maker. Instead of passing judgment, the judge issues a Proposal for Decision, which the board then votes to accept or reject.

The disciplinary options are the same whether there is a hearing or a settlement. In the most extreme cases, regulators may suspend a clinician's license for a period of months or years, or revoke it entirely. If the infraction is considered relatively minor—failure to renew a license on time, for instance— the board can take non-punitive administrative action that does not directly affect the clinician's license at all. Reprimands, usually involving a warning or letter of concern, are common, as are fines. Even though reprimands are less significant than license revocation or suspension, they are still formal disciplinary acts that become a matter of public record.

When the offense falls somewhere between these two extremes, as most do, the board or college may require the clinician to complete specific continuing education (CME, CE, etc.) courses, undergo treatment at a state or provincial/territorial physician health program or other professional health program (e.g., Nurses' Health Program), or take some other remedial step before being allowed to return to practice.

Rehabilitation is not an option a board offers lightly. Outside evaluators are often consulted first to determine if the clinician is likely to be helped by such measures, and once the program is completed, the clinician can be placed on probation for a period of time to help ensure that the rehabilitation has had more than a temporary impact.

Boards and regulatory colleges can also decide that a clinician should be allowed to return to practice, but only under certain conditions. The board may apply a restriction to the clinician's license or practice. It may require a clinician to use a chaperone at all times or to stop treating patients of a particular gender. A restricted license might mean the clinician can no longer prescribe controlled substances or perform certain procedures. Failure to abide by such requirements and restrictions can result in loss of license.

Being Disciplined By The Board Or Regulatory College

People who have lived through a tsunami often describe what at first seems an unremarkable line of water approaching. But the wall of water doesn't stop; it keeps coming, relentlessly uprooting everything that once seemed permanent and secure. The seemingly unending impacts that follow in the wake of serious professional discipline are like that. One occupational therapist in the US described it this way:

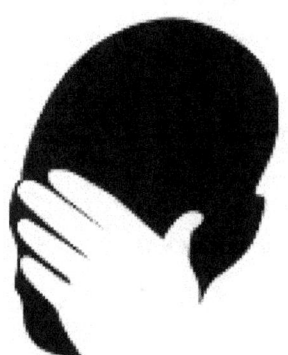

"After my license was suspended, I felt so ashamed I stopped going out in public. I had panic attacks. And while I didn't contemplate suicide, I prayed every night that God would take me. And I woke up each morning devastated that even He didn't think I was worth taking.

"My own physician prescribed an antidepressant, which offered some relief. I also went to see a counselor, but when the paychecks and health insurance stopped, I was forced to choose between the medication and the counseling. I chose the medication.

"I still had to earn a living so I took a series of low-level jobs. I was a clerk at a clothing store, a secretary for a local non-profit, and a waiter at a local country club—until someone recognized me and complained that I was not fit to work there. "The gift that keeps on taking," someone in

my remedial course told me."

When a complaint is made and your regulator opens an investigation, it can seem like a ludicrous overreaction. If you're the one being investigated, you may, like many, think it will all blow over or end up with a simple fine, like a parking ticket. For months, your life may go on as it always has, even as the case is passed to a probable-cause or Inquiries, Complaints, and Reports Committee and then onto the licensing board or college Disciplinary Committee.

But then the board or college announces its decision. It is not a parking ticket. Your license has been suspended or revoked; or perhaps you've been put on probation and told to enroll in remedial classes. You're in shock. "How can this be happening? It was a momentary mistake in a long, unblemished career. It doesn't make any sense."

Before you have a chance to regain your footing, the wave of devastation surges on, sweeping away the life you have known. Even a light disciplinary action—a six-month probation, say—can trigger almost immediate action by the rest of the medical credentialing community. Once a board in the US posts its decision on the National Practitioner Data Bank,[10] (where it will live forever), your hospital credentials are pulled, your board certification revoked, and your insurance protection is withdrawn. And as matters of public record, Canadian discipline committee decisions can be picked up by the news media and viewed by patients and regulators in other jurisdictions where you may be licensed. The career you have worked so hard to build now lies in rubble at your feet.

Anger is likely to be your first response. The board or college is just wrong, unjust. You will fight back, appeal, make this right. But sooner or later you learn that your outrage and resistance only make things worse. Eventually, you have to face the fact that no amount of fighting is going to change their decision. You have to accept the reality of what has happened.

And then it hits you: you are no longer the respected professional you have always known yourself to be. Colleagues, partners, patients, neighbors—nearly everyone you thought of as part of your life—now shun you, as if your shame is contagious. If you're lucky, your closest family and friends will stick with you, but you can see how they, too, are suffering as a result.

You feel humiliated, ashamed, and afraid to go out and risk the scorn of others who have heard about what's happened. And as the local media jumps on the story, the circle of those aware of your case grows exponentially. The mere possibility of meeting people at the mall brings on a panic attack. You start shopping in the middle of the night.

If you're like many professionals, you have come to define yourself by what you do, to equate your value as a human being with the respect and admiration your career has brought you. Now all that is gone.

Nothing feels secure anymore, not even your identity. Even if criminal charges are not filed, and you avoid jail, you will likely face legal fees and possible civil penalties. Your marriage may flounder. At this point, all the rage you had been directing outward—at the board/college, at the person who brought the complaint—turns inward.

Months of deep depression are common at this stage, leading many to contemplate suicide. A small number, though it's unclear how many, actually take their own lives. The vast majority of violators find the strength to seek help and move forward. For those who hang on, the crucial next step can seem the most degrading. With no source of income and bills piling up, once lavish lifestyles have to be abandoned. No longer able to do what they have always done, many are compelled to take whatever work they can find, however distasteful. A dental surgeon ends up selling cars; a psychiatrist answers phones; a psychologist drives for Uber and Lyft.

Recovering From A Violation

Some offenders, those the board believes capable of change, are given a second chance. Most end up reclaiming their careers, but the path they follow is no less harrowing. They typically pass through four distinct stages.

Stage 1: Denial

The first response to professional discipline is usually denial. Outraged by the situation they find themselves in, many deny that they have done anything wrong. They insist that no real harm was done and express amazement that the person even filed charges. Some go further, accusing those they have harmed with wanting to harm them. Whomever they blame, this stage ends with the inevitable realization that blaming others is a dead end and the only way forward is to accept responsibility.

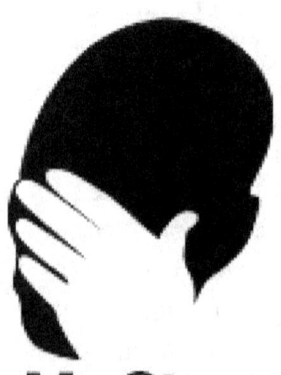

My Story

"At first I was angry and hurt. I felt that I had been wronged by the system and blamed everyone but myself—my patient, the prosecutor, the board. Eventually, through therapy and insight, I was able to let go of the anger and get past who was at fault. The critical piece for me was to realize that what I had done was, in fact, a boundary infraction. I came to see how I had strayed outside the professional boundaries that are meant to protect both the patient and the physician."

Stage 2: Victim Empathy

Once they have stopped feeling victimized themselves, offenders must begin to focus on the person they have victimized. Many boundary violators insist that no one has been hurt by their actions. The most they will admit to is violating a rule—a far cry from acknowledging that they have genuinely hurt a vulnerable patient.

There are many reasons people resist acknowledging their victim's pain. One of the most significant is a fear of losing a long-held and often unrealistic image of themselves as noble healers. People are also afraid of the guilt they'll feel.

But it's not until they overcome these inhibitions and empathize with their victim, come to understand the real pain they have caused, that offenders can fully accept responsibility for their violation. Before returning a clinician to practice, regulators generally want to know that they have reached this point—and with good reason.

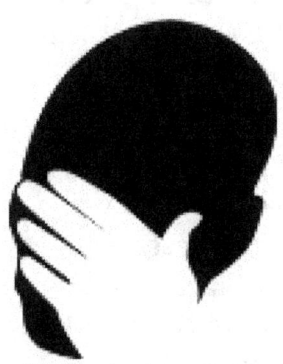

Only someone who truly understands the pain they have caused can be trusted to avoid causing it again.

"At first, I felt like something was happening to me rather than because of me. But I went to see a therapist and eventually realized that I had injured a good person. It was terribly painful. I'm not by nature a hurtful person. I've wanted to be a nurse since I was ten, and I've loved being a smart, helpful nurse practitioner. The knowledge that I had hurt someone who came to me for help was excruciat-

ing. I felt very guilty and depressed about what I had done to my patient, to my profession, and to my family."

Stage Three: Rock Bottom

For those who hang on and allow themselves to empathize with their victim, the crucial next stage can seem the most depressing.

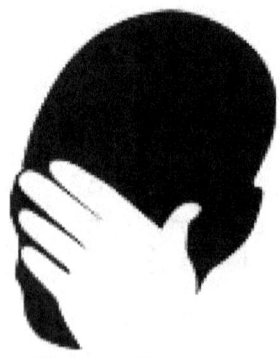
My Story

"The financial impact didn't hit me right away. But the emotional impact did and it was far worse. Health care had been my life and now it was gone. Even more painful, I had always thought of myself as a good person, someone who cared more for others, particularly my patients, than for myself. Now I was being told that I wasn't fit to be around patients. I didn't know who I was anymore or what I was going to do."

This deep level of depression leads many to seek escape through alcohol or drugs. Some commit suicide.

Support is crucial at this point, both from professionals and from others who are facing, or who have faced, similar situations. The testimony of those who have fought their way through the same darkness, and those who have helped them, offers proof that there is hope. One physician who enrolled in PBI's weekly supportive teleconference described the faculty-guided sessions as her lifeline to the rest of the world. "The others were understanding, supportive and sometimes helpfully challenging. As the weeks and months rolled by, it began to sink in that I was not the only one going through this. I was not alone."

Stage Four: Reinvention

Now comes the difficult work of rebuilding a life and possibly a career. You can't fix yourself if you don't understand what's broken, so the clinician now has to do what few are able to accomplish without help—question their most basic assumptions about who they are, what they are good at, and what gives their life meaning and purpose. Answering these questions leads to radical recalibration.

People who complete this phase do not simply return to their previous life. They create new ways of living and working that reflect what they have learned about their own frailties and strengths. Having been forced to try something other than the career that has always defined them, they can begin to take stock of who they are and what they have to offer as unique individuals, not simply as healthcare professionals. Having lost so much of what they thought was essential, they find new freedom to rethink priorities and reinvent themselves.

They may change the kind of medicine they practice or the kinds of patients they treat. They will almost certainly devote more attention to family and friends outside of work so they can assign appropriate attention to those they care for professionally. Almost always, those who reach this point begin a journey that brings them not back to where they were, but to someplace better, leaving them more balanced, more secure, and many say happier than they were before their regulator sanctioned them.

Having come so far, the rehabilitated clinician can lose it all if they fail to embrace humility. They have to accept themselves for who they are, flaws and all. As they return to work, they must remain alert for warning signs they might have missed in the past and be willing to seek the help they once viewed as weakness.

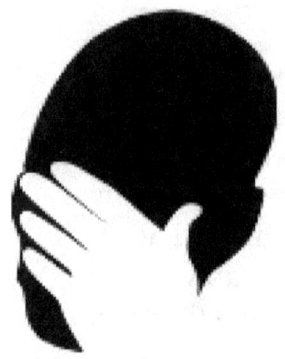

My Story

"Facing up to what I had done totally changed my sense of who I was. I finally understood what it meant to be human. I had grown up trying to be the perfect child my parents expected me to be. That's why I was always such a straight arrow. But now I realized that I had an internal life, like everyone else, and just as much need of companionship as others have.

I had been working way too hard, seeing more patients than I should have, serving on committees, teaching classes, often going without eating or sleeping enough. And all this work had left me with no time for personal relationships. I was very busy and very lonely, which was perhaps one reason I responded as I did to a patient who seemed warm and understanding.

This change in how I saw myself opened me up to a fuller understanding of other people. As I realized what I was going through, I realized more and more that others were going through their own troubles. This has made me, I think, a much better clinician because now I can understand the pain others go through in a very profound way.

I am also taking much better care of myself. Now that I know what can happen if I work too hard, I have made personal time with family and friends a priority. I still sometimes feel guilty about neglecting my patients, but I am more realistic now about how much work is too much for me."

Takeaways

- Maintaining your patients' trust is your primary professional obligation and a condition of your licensure.

- Some boundaries are explicitly defined in law. Keeping up with state or provincial law is as important as keeping up with the latest research.

- Boundaries governing the clinician-patient relationship are open to board or regulatory college interpretation. State/provincial law allows regulators to make case-by-case decisions.

- Any non-medical "dual relationship" with a patient jeopardizes your clinical objectivity.

- There is no such thing as consensual sex between a clinician and a patient.

- You are responsible for managing your relationship with your patients, regardless of their behavior or motivations.

- The regulator's duty is to protect the public, not you.

- Your license to practice is a privilege, not a right. The board/college that granted your license can take it away.

- In any dispute, the board/college is far more likely to side with the patient.

- Board/college discipline or sanction often triggers a seemingly endless period of disruption, sweeping away everything you thought permanent and secure.

- Some offenders are given a second chance. The path they follow is no less harrowing than the one followed by those less fortunate.

> # The Four Laws of Professional Boundaries
>
> Everyone has a violation potential which is constantly changing.
>
> Perception is 9/10 of the law.
>
> Protect yourself at all times.
>
> The board (or college) decides what's right, not you.

Resources

Find your state medical board's website
https://www.fsmb.org/contact-a-state-medical-board/

Find Your Provincial Or Territorial Medical Board's Website

fmrac.ca/members/

HIPAA for Professionals
https://www.hhs.gov/hipaa/for-professionals/index.html

Provincial And Territorial Privacy Laws And Oversight

https://www.priv.gc.ca/en/about-the-opc/what-we-do/provincial-and-territorial-collaboration/provincial-and-territorial-privacy-laws-and-oversight/

What You Need To Know About Hipaa And Canada Health Information Privacy

- Compares privacy laws in both countries, including the location of storage of protected information and province-by-province differences

https://vsee.com/blog/hipaa-canada-health-information-privacy/#:~:text=What%20are%20the%20rules%20in,HIPAA)%20in%20the%20United%20States.

Medicare Fraud & Abuse: Prevent, Detect, Report https://www.cms.gov/Outreach-and-Education/Medicare-Learning-Network-MLN/MLNProducts/Downloads/Fraud-Abuse-MLN4649244.pdf

[1]

PART 2:
How Good Clinicians Get Into Trouble

The Insidious Process Leading to a Violation

○ Forces Pushing You Towards a Violation

○ Warning Signs

Clinicians' attitudes towards professional boundaries often reflect what they've learned about personal boundaries. The process begins early in life. Small children test personal boundaries as they work to figure out their relationship to the world around them and how to handle new, powerful emotions. They are teasing out just how far they can go, and how far they want to go.

When parents set and enforce clear boundaries, they teach their children something important about their place in the world: "Your power has limits and there are times when you have to restrain yourself to accommodate others." Toddlers may feel angry and resentful at first, but once the tantrum fades, they feel safer and less anxious knowing there are adults who will set limits that keep them safe and help them manage those overwhelming feelings. Such testing continues throughout childhood and adolescence.

Older children and teens learn a great deal about boundaries by watching their parents. If parents always put their own needs first, their children are unlikely to learn the value of setting boundaries for themselves when their own interests conflict with others. At the other end of the spectrum, parents who always put others' needs ahead of their own fail to teach their children how to set personal boundaries that protect them from others' intrusive demands.

The situation is seldom so simple, of course. And as important as early testing and parental models are, we never stop learning about boundaries. If we're lucky, our understanding matures as we age. We learn how to respect others' boundaries and how to set boundaries for ourselves. We learn, too, that static, rigid boundaries can be as unhelpful as boundaries that are too amorphous and elastic. Healthy boundaries, like healthy cell membranes, regulate effectively by responding dynamically to changing environments.

Those who don't learn these lessons in their personal lives are more likely to have difficulty with professional boundaries. The insecure adult who has never learned to say "no" becomes the clinician who is more interested in pleasing her patients than using her own best clinical judgment. The adolescent who learned to manipulate others for his own ends becomes the predatory clinician who misuses his power over vulnerable patients.

Many clinicians learn the wrong lessons on the job. Even the best adjusted professional, with a mature grasp of personal boundaries, does not enter the profession with a clear understanding of professional boundaries. The clinician-patient relationship is unlike other relationships and the responsible clinician must learn the unique boundaries that govern it. Unfortunately, the subject is given scant attention in professional school. For the most part, clinicians learn about professional boundaries in much the same way they learned about personal boundaries growing up, by observing how others behave.

Needless to say, it is difficult to learn the importance of establishing and respecting boundaries when those around you routinely disregard them. Harder still when schools, hospitals and private practices shy away from disciplining even flagrant violators, especially if they are a source of significant revenue for the institution.

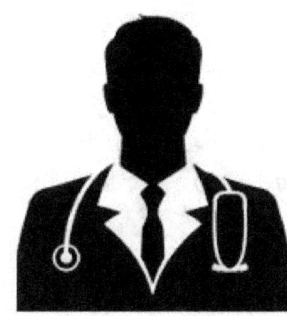

As head of cardiology at a prestigious medical school, Dr. Byron was admired for his research and the millions of dollars in funding it attracted. When he made advances towards Susan, a researcher on his team, the young woman was not surprised. Dr. Byron had a reputation. She did become concerned when he persisted even after she had rebuffed him several times. When the administration failed to take her complaints seriously, Susan decided she'd had enough and found a position at another university.

Her husband, however, stayed on after being promised a promotion. But the moment Susan was gone, Dr. Byron went after her husband. He vetoed his expected promotion and interfered with the publication of an important research paper.

This time the charges were too egregious to ignore. A university committee investigated the situation and formally recommended that Dr. Byron be terminated. Even so, the

> well-known and well-funded professor was only briefly suspended and allowed to continue as head of a major research center at the school. And although he lost his endowed chair, a few years later he was honored with another.

It's impossible to judge how common such situations are, since many cases are buried or settled with as little publicity as possible. But it's not only major incidents like this one that influence what young clinicians learn about appropriate and inappropriate behavior. A recent survey in the U.K. revealed that medical students frequently witnessed their instructors behaving in ways they knew were inappropriate.

"Some of the testimonies gathered from medical students are jaw-dropping," noted a BBC report on the survey. One patient was told by a physician, "You shouldn't even be here. You're so fat I shouldn't even have considered you for surgery." In another instance, a physician called out to a female student, "You there, the decoration, why did you even come to med school? Do you have a brain in your pretty head?"

"Students pick up these subtle patterns of behavior and they come to learn this is how things are done around here, this is how work is done," Dr. Lynn Monrouxe of Cardiff University told the BBC. "The small subtle interactions that happen day in, day out—not necessarily the big, shocking, news-grabbing headlines—It's the things that can't be counted that really count."[11]

The Insidious Process Leading To A Violation

When asked how he went bankrupt, Mike Campbell, a character in Ernest Hemingway's 1926 novel *The Sun Also Rises* answers, "Two ways. Gradually, then suddenly." That's how medical careers end, too. Boundary violations don't just happen. They often begin imperceptibly and progress slowly enough to avoid detection—until it's too late.

The first phase is usually a passing thought or fantasy about a patient. These are common. And while some fantasies are sexual, many are not. One physical therapist daydreams about hanging out with a friendly patient. A dentist thinks about asking an attorney/patient for legal advice. The fantasy may even be altruistic: "I can't solve all of Mary's financial problems, but I can at least lend her cab fare home..." These kinds of thoughts are considered "drifts," and as long as they remain thoughts rather than actions, they are generally considered harmless.

But there are times when "drifts" lead to something more —either a "crossing" or a "violation." The difference between the two is supposed to be that a violation causes harm, whereas a crossing does not. But the distinction is not all that helpful, because it's often unclear whether or not harm has been done. If you offer to pay for a lab test that a financially stressed patient can't afford, have you done any harm?

What if the patient is so mortified by your offer that they fail to get the test or keep their next appointment and ends up at the ER a week later?

There is rarely a clear, definable moment when a harmless drift slips into the dangerous territory of a crossing or violation. As the following case illustrates, the path from one to the other is less a straight line than a slippery slope.

> *Dr. Allison Garfield had been treating Fred for diabetes for over a year. During that time, she had come to enjoy his visits. Fred, who had started out quite anxious about his health, found Dr. Garfield's calm manner and friendly*

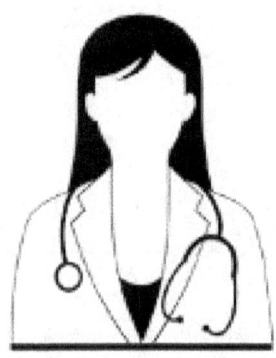

Case File

banter comforting. As time went on, he began complimenting the doctor on her expertise, as well as her stylish clothes. Not wanting to disrupt what she felt was a strong doctor-patient relationship, she playfully parried his lighthearted flirtation.

When they met by chance one morning at the local coffee shop, Fred invited her to join him and they ended up talking for almost an hour. In the course of the conversation, Fred mentioned that he and his wife were having problems.

The next time Fred came into the office, he was the last patient of the day, and the routine 15-minute visit lasted well after the office had officially closed and the staff had gone home. Doctor and patient walked out to their cars together and lingered in the parking lot, talking and laughing for a long time. Nothing more happened that night, but for the next several weeks Dr. Garfield made a habit of seeing Fred at the end of the day, and the scene was repeated more than once.

Finally, one evening a few months later, the two ended up together in Fred's car, and then at his house. His wife was out of town, and doctor and patient spent the night together.

When Dr. Garfield awoke in the morning, she realized what she had done and left hastily. She tried to pull back but Fred kept calling her at work and emailing her. When he told her he loved her, she said she would have to stop seeing him and referred him to another *doctor in town.*

Hurt and angry, Fred told his wife what had happened and she complained to the board. Dr. Garfield's license was revoked.

It may be a cliché, but the concept of the slippery slope is useful: once you realize how easily minor mistakes can lead to serious consequences, you are far more likely to notice when you've stepped too close to the edge. (You'll find warning signs to watch for in Chapter 4.)

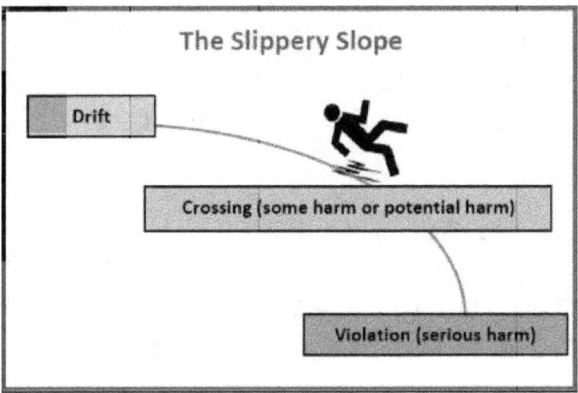

The Forces
Pushing You Towards a Violation

No matter how sure-footed you are, it is difficult to avoid a career-ending violation without a firm understanding of the forces working against you. The more you know about these challenges, the better prepared you will be to keep your footing.

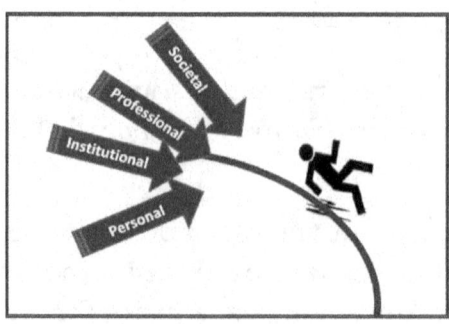

Societal challenges

Social Media. The ubiquity of social media poses a serious challenge for all clinicians. As both clinicians and patients share thoughts and stories on Facebook, Instagram, Snapchat and other social media platforms, dangers proliferate, including:

- Saying too much: People tend to lose normal inhibitions online, and end up saying things they would never say in person. And once you say something online, you lose control of it—forever.

- Not knowing who you're talking to: When you send emails and texts, you don't know who has access to them on the other end.

- Crossing state or provincial/territorial or national lines: Clinical advice you offer online can be read or passed along to people in other jurisdictions. If you're not licensed in those jurisdictions, you can be charged with practicing without a license.

- Losing control of your staff: Like the captain of a ship, you are responsible for your staff's actions. If a staff member posts a photo or comment that violates the law, you're the one who will be disciplined.

- Becoming too chummy with patents: A 2011 legal

decision established that physicians who share too much personal information with patients online are implicitly inviting them to get closer than is professionally appropriate.[12]

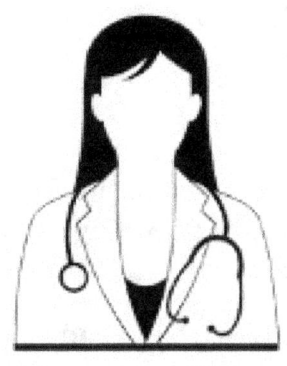

Case File

After a long day in the OR, Dr. Granger, an orthopedic surgeon, liked to unwind in online chat rooms. He never used his real name and enjoyed the anonymity of his online persona. When people complained about medical problems, Dr. Granger sometimes offered advice after mentioning he was an experienced physician.

When women in one chat room became flirtatious, the surgeon ended up sexting with some of them individually. Eventually, a few of the women compared experiences and discovered they were not the only ones Dr. Granger was sexting. They were outraged at having been manipulated and complained to the medical board. In particular, the women claimed Dr. Granger had played up his medical experience to elicit intimate details. After an investigation, board members disciplined the surgeon for using his medical license to exploit the women. He was suspended for three months and put on probation for a year.

Electronic communication. Texts and emails have become so common, it's easy to forget that they carry significant risks, including:

- Violating HIPAA or PIPEDA rules: Because HIPAA and PIPEDA give individuals the right to access and amend protected health information, you have to document any information you acquire or send over the internet. It's also important to password protect any information on electronic devices and use HIPAA- or PI-

PEDA-compliant software.

- <u>Creating unrealistic expectations</u>: Answering patient questions on a personal cell phone, especially outside of regular office hours, can raise expectations that you will always be available at that number. If you're not, the patient may well file a complaint.

- <u>Helping the prosecution</u>: Lawyers will tell you, the "e" in email stands for evidence. Most of the texts and emails that show up in court are not the reason for the case but rather evidence supporting the charges.

Cultural Diversity. Clinicians in both the U.S. and Canada are far more likely to see patients from other cultures than they were 20 or 30 years ago. Patients in both countries are increasingly likely to be treated by physicians from other cultures, as more than 25% of physicians and surgeons in both the U.S. and Canada are currently foreign born. Because of this diversity, patients and clinicians sometimes bring very different cultural assumptions to their professional relationship.

<u>Clinicians caring for patients from other cultures</u>. Patients from some cultures may find the behavior of U.S. physicians cold and impersonal. Other patients, whose religion restricts interaction between unrelated members of the opposite sex, may find routine physical exams not just offensive, but frightening.

> *Zara had been Dr. Bruce Phillips 'patient for several months. A recent immigrant from the Middle East,*
>
> *she was always accompanied by her husband. In fact, for the first few visits Zara and her husband, Sameer, insisted that the physician address his questions to Sameer. Over time, Zara joined the conversation and Dr. Phillips felt*

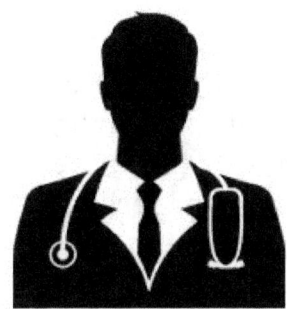

they had developed a solid professional relationship.

One day Sameer was unable to join his wife for her regular visit. As he always did, Dr. Phillips was careful to explain to Zara what he was doing during the physical exam, and she did not protest. But when her husband found out that she had been touched when he was not present, he was insulted and outraged. He filed charges of sexual assault and told the board that his wife felt violated by the routine exam. Dr. Phillips was put on probation and required to take a course in cultural sensitivity.

Whatever the cultural differences are between you and your patient, you as the clinician are responsible for managing the relationship. This is equally true for domestically-trained clinicians treating patients from other cultures and foreign-trained clinicians treating patients in their home country.

Foreign-born clinicians caring for patients in North America. Some clinicians from other cultures are accustomed to a level of personal interaction—whether it be physical contact or topics of conversation—that both patients and regulators find inappropriate. For example, in many parts of the Middle East, Latin America, Africa, and southern Europe, people are far more comfortable with physical contact than most Americans and Canadians are, especially in a medical setting. One Latin American physician who had been practicing in the U.S. for years without incident hugged a female patient who he thought needed comforting. Having done the same thing many times before, he was astonished when the woman claimed that he touched her breast, and then filed a complaint.

In another case, a Middle Eastern surgeon had routinely hugged nurses he worked with as a way of saying thank you. When he began practicing in North America, many of his coworkers tolerated his expressions of gratitude. But several female nurses felt uncomfortable and resisted what they considered improper touching. When the surgeon continued the practice, apparently oblivious to their discomfort, they filed charges.

Other clinicians new to the U.S. or Canada treat virtually all their patients, especially those from their own culture, as if they were relatives. Whether they are members of a close-knit Hispanic neighborhood or a first-generation Korean community, these clinicians tend to have trouble saying no to people they regard as brothers and sisters. Rather than risk seeming rude, clinicians in such situations have loaned patients large sums of money, put them up in their homes, accepted gifts, and offered them employment—all against the explicit policies of the office they worked in.

Doctors trained in a hierarchical society may have the opposite problem. Fifty years ago patients and staff in the U.S. were expected to accept the authority of physicians and to follow their instructions without question. Today, patients often come to appointments with information they have gathered online, ready to participate in any decisions about their care. And staff are generally encouraged to voice concerns and share opinions.

Physicians trained elsewhere often react to this collaborative culture much as a physician from 1950 would; they are outraged. They feel disrespected by patients who ask questions and raise concerns and sometimes react angrily to what they consider a lack of appropriate deference. The problem can be even more pronounced in interactions with colleagues—nurses and other medical professionals

—whom these doctors tend to treat dismissively, if not with overt hostility. Needless to say, such behavior leads to complaints and often to disciplinary action.

Institutional Challenges

Some hospitals support their staff's efforts to maintain professional boundaries, but many turn a blind eye to offenses. And there are those that actively, even if unintentionally, encourage violations (then quickly back away when there are repercussions). Many of these institutional challenges can be traced back to financial pressures.

Patients as customers. With 30% of a U.S. hospital's Medicare reimbursement now based on patient- satisfaction surveys, hospitals increasingly view patients as customers and pressure physicians and nurses to do all they can to keep them happy. In 2021, the Canadian Institute for Health Information will begin publicly reporting five measures from the Canadian Patient Experiences Survey on Inpatient Care on a facility level as part of its work on health system performance measurement.

To ensure customer satisfaction, and earn high marks on those surveys, some hospitals encourage doctors and nurses to "go the extra mile" to please patients, all too often without regard to maintaining appropriate professional behavior. Others reinforce the message by tying financial bonuses to patient satisfaction scores. Practitioners in these institutions may be coached to offer anxious patients a reassuring pat on the back or a quick hug — never mind the alarming prevalence of sexual abuse in our culture and the risk that a previously traumatized patient will misinterpret the physical contact.

Conflicting demands for productivity. Like all corporate enterprises, today's health care establishment seeks to increase productivity, which for clinicians generally means less time with each patient and less time for empathy. Those who struggle to maintain an emotional connection with patients despite the challenges risk compassion fatigue. "When the workload is heavy and there's not enough time to address all the issues that are occurring," says Funmilayo Rachal, a board-certified adult and forensic psychiatrist, "a physician can definitely get overwhelmed and develop burnout."[13] Others retreat behind a wall of professional aloofness to avoid being overwhelmed.

Ironically, the same corporate mentality that impedes empathy is also fueling a resurgence of interest in how clinicians can better relate to patients. Empathy, it turns out, is good for business. Research has shown that physician empathy boosts patient compliance, positive outcomes, and patient satisfaction—all considered "key performance indicators" at the corporate level.

Caught in the middle—between the empathy-dampening demand for productivity and the business-driven interest in increasing empathy—are physicians, nurses, and all the other medical professionals trying to care for patients in the world of 21st-century health care.

Lack of safeguards. The best way to avoid potentially disastrous misunderstandings is to have another person in the room who can help clear things up on the spot or help resolve "he said-she said" controversies after the fact. But hospitals facing crushing financial burdens are often loathe to provide the staffing needed to ensure the presence of a medical chaperone. (For more on chaperones, see Part 3: Best Practices.)

The absence of a chaperone makes a clinician's notes all the more crucial, especially when it's the patient who behaves inappropriately. But there are hospitals, wary of offending patients, that discourage doctors from noting such incidents in the patient's chart. That not only puts other practitioners treating the patient at a disadvantage, it also deprives the current physician of valuable protection.

> *The first time Doris playfully slapped Dr. Greely on the butt, he was too surprised to say anything. But when she did it again, he stopped and asked her to please stop. Doris tried to laugh it off, but Dr. Greely asked her how she would feel if the situation was reversed. She laughed again and said that would be fine, but the physician could see that she was embarrassed and angry.*

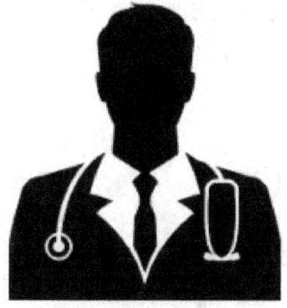

Case File

> *Dr. Greely had been reprimanded in the past for noting things in patients' charts that might embarrass them, so he did not mention the incident in his notes. When Doris told the patient liaison representative that it was the doctor who had patted her inappropriately, there was no way for Dr. Greely to corroborate his version of events.*
>
> *Fortunately for him, Doris did not press the matter any further, but a disciplinary note was added to the physician's personnel record.*

<u>Blaming physicians.</u> Hospitals often avoid censure by firing clinicians charged with a violation, even if the hospital itself had unofficially sanctioned the offending behavior. A hospital that tolerates an offensive senior practitioner will generally express outrage when a patient files a complaint. And when there are a string of incidents at a hospital, most institutions will respond by "cleaning house," rather than accepting responsibility and considering how the organizational culture might be

fostering problems.

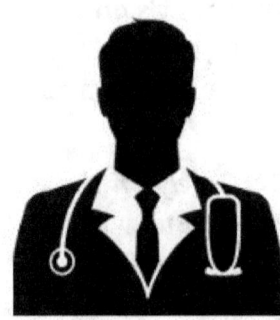

Case File

Orthopedic surgeons were important to the Crittlebrook Hospital, but several of the most experienced physicians were losing time at work because of back problems. When an anaesthesiologist provided pain relief to one of the surgeons so he could keep on working, others began asking for similar help. Word got back to hospital administrators, but they did not interfere with the clearly inappropriate practice.

Eventually, a hospital inspection uncovered what was going on. Concerned about losing its accreditation, the hospital terminated the anaesthesiologist, who then lost his license.

Professional Challenges

<u>Challenging patients.</u> General practitioners often end up treating patients who should be seen by specialists. But the reality is that psychiatric patients are now more likely to be seen by general practitioners than by psychiatrists, and patients with chronic pain are more often treated by a primary care practitioner than by a pain specialist. This is risky both for the patient, who may be receiving sub-optimal care, and for the clinician, who is venturing into a world of boundary issues they know little about. (See <u>Part 3: Best Practices</u>.)

<u>Patients with personal problems.</u> For all their education and training, healthcare professionals are often surprisingly naïve. They lose sight of the fact that patients have lives and problems they don't always share with their clinician. People who come in with sinusitis or a sprained ankle may well have been sexually traumatized at some

point in their lives, may be suffering through wrenching personal problems or struggling with mental health issues. These stresses can influence a patient's reactions in unexpected ways.

Electronic health records. One of the most common problems with EHR systems is the auto-populate feature: you hit a button and a bunch of fields are filled in. One physician was shocked to discover that his records showed him giving every one of his patients, male and female, a breast exam. Regulators are sensitized to this problem. If they start seeing the same exact information in patients' records over and over again, they are going to start asking questions.

The struggle with power. Patients aren't the only ones vulnerable to a healthcare professional's power. Clnicians themselves often fall victim to the power inherent in their position. Some are seduced by the authority and prestige that comes with wearing a white coat. Others are so uncomfortable with their own power they seek to escape it. The two responses may seem worlds apart, but they lead to similar results—none of them good.

Aside from sociopaths who abuse patients without hesitation or remorse—and tend to make the headlines—physicians and other clinicians don't generally make a conscious decision to misuse their power. Instead, boundary violations generally arise unnoticed as these clinicians respond in various ways to the power society (and patients) confer on them. While every clinician's response to power is individual, many of those who struggle with the issue fall into one of three categories:

> **The Entitled Clinician.** The first time young doctors ceremoniously don white coats during graduation, they are likely to feel both elated and honored, not to

mention nervous and even intimidated by their new role. Over time, these feelings change, of course. Most clinicians gain the self-confidence they need to get the job done without losing an appreciation of all the job demands.

But for some, the years they spend healing the sick and winning accolades alter their perception of themselves. They stop viewing their profession as an honor and come to see themselves as professionals to be honored. Humility gives way to hubris. Most of these people are smart, accomplished clinicians, but with experience and age comes a dangerous sense of entitlement.

For them, the white coat becomes something much grander over time, a kind of royal garment that endows them not only with a sense of infallibility but also of invulnerability that is out of touch with reality. Eventually, the cautious concern that guided them in their youth is replaced by impatience with rules and regulations. As professional arrogance takes over, the risk of recklessness increases, both in terms of personal and medical judgment.

Peter Pronovost, MD, Ph.D., whose promotion of medical checklists saved thousands of lives, believes that arrogant doctors who place too much trust in their own judgment are a leading cause of preventable medical errors, from which thousands die every year. "Physicians are overconfident about the quality of care they provide, believing things will go right rather than wrong, assuming they provide higher-quality care than the evidence suggests, and thinking they alone have sufficient knowledge and skills to provide care," Pronovost wrote in a JAMA editorial.[14]

The same arrogance leads to boundary violations, as clinicians place more and more faith in their own decision-making and feel less and less accountable to external judgment. As they achieve seniority, they see themselves as having outgrown the professional boundaries that define their role.

The Distant Clinician. In her book, *At Personal Risk*, Marilyn R. Peterson describes a fundamental tension at the core of doctors' professional lives. Physicians are continually expected to weigh the available evidence and make critical decisions based on calculated risks—often with one eye on the clock and the other on the budget, frequently with patients, families and administrators looking over their shoulder. And they are supposed to do all this while projecting the calm certainty patients crave. Yet these same doctors often feel unsure of themselves, uncertain about their own judgment, and all too dependent on forces beyond their control—the labs they use, the hospitals they work for, the insurance companies that pay them, even the imperfect science they rely on.

This tension between the myth of the all-knowing health professional and the reality of the fallible human being in a white coat, between the reality of power and the feeling of powerlessness, is unavoidable. But for many clinicians, it is also intolerable. These practitioners try to ease the strain, says Peterson, in one of two ways. The Distant Physician tries to strengthen their sense of control by seeing their patients not as people in pain but as cases to be solved. Compassion and empathy are dismissed as emotional distractions that interfere with scientific objectivity. Peterson sums up the danger implicit in this attitude:

> "Divorcing parts of ourselves allow us to divorce the comparable parts of the client. By canceling out our own and the client's personhood, we, in effect, dismiss the relevance of the interpersonal connection. From this vantage point, we are vulnerable to denying you personal responsibility for the emotional impact of our actions on others... With less room for the client, the danger that we will misuse our power increases."[15]

The Familiar Clinician takes the opposite approach. In an effort to escape her discomfort with the power she wields over patients, she shies away from taking charge and making decisions. Rather than holding herself aloof from her patients, this clinician pulls up a chair and chats with them as equals. She views her power over them "as non-existent or irrelevant," to quote a recent research study that explored physicians' perceptions of their own power.

> "These physicians describe how they are on a level playing field with patients, which they emphasize has the essence of a collegial and friendly relationship. One physician captured the notion that his interactions with patients were situated in a flat hierarchical power structure in the following quotation: "A lot of patients really want to be an equal partner in the learning. And some of them are very intelligent and they will ask you difficult questions. And that's fine, I kind of like that."[16]

This abdication of professional responsibility can lead not only to poor medical decisions— influenced by what the patient wants, not what they need—but also to boundary violations. The failure to take charge is essentially a refusal to set limits, to establish the boundaries that create a safe space between the vulnerable patient and the clinician responsible for the relationship. Simply denying the power differential between clinician and patient does not, of course, alter the reality of the clinician's superior position. It does, however, undermine her focus on exercising restraint and staying within bounds. With little power comes little responsibility.

Personal Challenges

<u>The demands of the job.</u> One of the defining challenges of a career in health care is making time for a personal life. Too often, clinicians feel forced to choose between providing quality care for patients and spending time with family and friends. It can be even harder to take time for yourself. With patients waiting for your help, it's all too easy to view "alone time" or a backyard barbecue as mere self-indulgence. Yet without such respites from work, the chronic stress of caring for others is simply unsustainable.

<u>Lack of self-care.</u> Clinicians tend to ignore the stress in their lives. The strain of constantly dealing with illness, pain, and death is difficult enough, and is often compounded by severe time constraints and a heavy load of paperwork. Healthcare professionals are also notoriously negligent about caring for themselves in general, and often fear the stigma of acknowledging and seeking help for mental health problems. The result:

- Physicians suffer a higher rate of addiction than the general population. According to a 2014 article in USA Today, across the U.S., more than 100,000 doctors, nurses, technicians, and other health professionals struggle with abuse or addiction.

- Physicians are at least as susceptible to depression as anyone else, probably more so (under- reporting makes it difficult to say for sure). Residents' rate of depression is more than twice the national average.

- Physicians report the highest burnout rate of all professions—46%, up from 42% just a couple of years ago.

- Physicians are at a much higher risk of dying from suicide than the general population.[17] In Canada, physicians have the highest rate of suicide of any profession, and double the rate compared with the general population.

<u>The role-vacuum.</u> Such over-investment in work is a major factor in burnout. It is also a primary driver of serious boundary violations. As overwhelming as they might be, frustration and fatigue are not the fundamental problems here. "The classic problem with the over-extended, overworked physician is that they lose connection to other relationship domains: friendship, intimacy, social involvement," explains Peter Graham, co-founder of Acumen Assessments and Acumen Institute and a specialist at assessing and treating boundary violators. "When those other relationship domains empty out what you get is a vacuum, what I call a role-vacuum, and that vacuum gets filled up with patients and co-workers."[18] Graham's comment applies to other clinicians just as much.

The consequences of this role-vacuum can vary. One nurse tries to fill the growing void in her personal life by devoting herself entirely to her patients. Anguished by their suffering, she works longer and longer hours attempting to ease their pain. Eventually, the constant emotional strain leads to "compassion fatigue." She ends up feeling exhausted and hopeless—burnt out.

THE PHYSICIAN'S GUIDE TO PROFESSIONAL BOUNDARIES

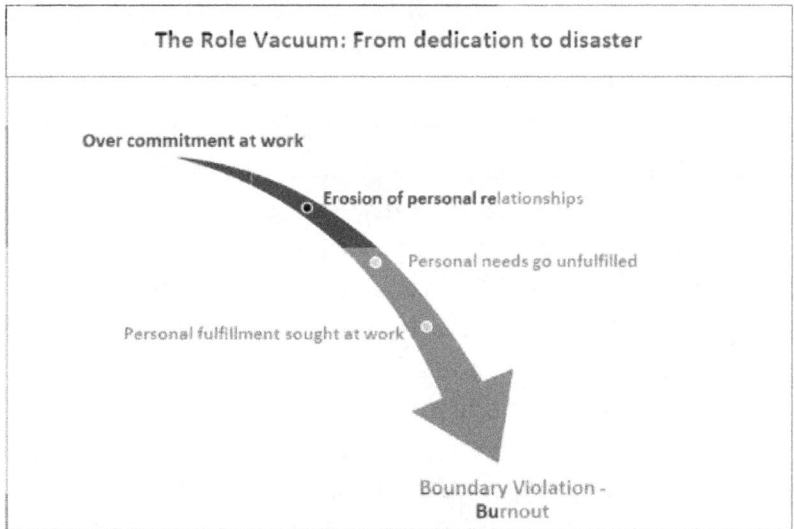

A physical therapist follows the same path to begin with, seeking comfort in his work with patients. But his over-involvement takes a different turn. Instead of burning out, he is energized by the adulation of those he cares for. Before long, he begins to find in the examining room the emotional connection he no longer finds at home. His path leads to an inappropriate relationship with a patient.

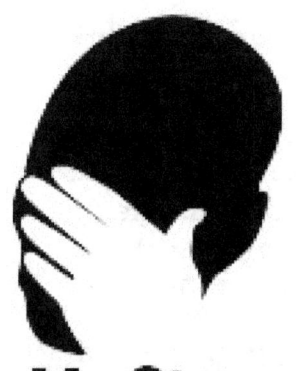

"It was just an innocent drink. The scans for Joan's little boy showed we were finally making progress after nearly losing him a year earlier. We were both so glad to hear the news, I honestly don't remember which of us suggested we celebrate at the wine bar down the block. But the office had closed, I was both exhausted and elated, and it felt cruel to just send Joan off into the night by herself. I may have hesitated a moment before agreeing to a drink, but when I thought about what was waiting for me at home, the choice seemed all too clear.

79

My wife had been complaining about my long hours for months. She had gotten so angry and bitter, it seemed we hardly talked anymore. I tried to smooth things over, but I'm a pediatric oncologist, and helping save children's lives is not just a nine to five commitment. Still, I did my best to separate my troubles at home from my problems at work. But that just left me feeling isolated, and my wife told me that simply coming home at a more reasonable hour was no answer if I came home distracted and distant.

So going out for a drink with someone who truly valued what I did and wanted to celebrate our success—well, it seemed like a nice thing to do."

Still others, unable to recharge their batteries outside the office, become overwhelmed by the constant strain of patient care. Exhausted, they find themselves simply going through the motions, moving from patient to patient and plowing through paperwork with less and less sense of purpose. Eventually, they feel used up, unappreciated and uncared for by anyone, at home or at work. Their burnout may lead to depression and even thoughts of suicide.

Or these same benumbed caregivers, no longer able to suppress the anger they feel at being taken for granted, explode in rage at staff, make inappropriate comments to patients, or try to self-medicate by writing themselves prescriptions for drugs that can help dull the pain.

What lies at the heart of all these potentially career-ending outcomes, whether burnout or boundary violation, is a failure to cultivate an identity outside of work, to create healthy boundaries between one's personal and professional lives.

<u>Hot and cold ethics</u>. Not all personal challenges can be

boiled down to an imbalance between personal and professional identities. Each of us has internal needs that drive us in ways we understand and many we don't. Remember the [Boundary Sphere illustration from earlier](#)? It's not enough to recognize the boundaries that define the sphere, you also have to come to terms with the internal forces that push you towards success—forces that, if unrestrained, can cause you to go too far.

The fact is, despite your extensive training, you are subject to the same forces of irrationality as every other human being. It doesn't matter how well you intellectually understand the professional boundaries involved in a case. Cool, rational analysis is no match for the pressures that build up in the heat of the moment. And those pressures are almost always the result of personal issues you don't fully understand or even acknowledge to yourself. Identifying these internal needs and fears is never easy and coming to terms with them is likely to be one of the most difficult personal challenges you face. It is also one of the most important things you can do to protect yourself, your career and your patients.

Warning Signs

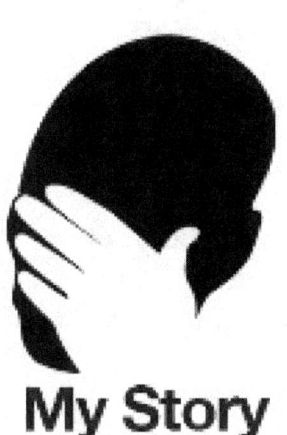

"I didn't know why, but I felt drawn to Beth during her first visit to the clinic. Nothing happened: I took her history, ordered some labs and told her to schedule a follow-up. A few weeks later, after I had seen her in the office a couple more times, she invited me to be her friend on Facebook. I don't usually communicate with patients on social media, but the request seemed harmless enough, so I agreed. I

started learning things about Beth's private life, especially her deteriorating relationship with a boyfriend. The next time she called and asked for an appointment, I agreed to stay late to accommodate her schedule. As soon as I closed the door, she burst into tears. I asked her if she was ok, and she started telling me all about her personal life. I listened and tried to help her calm down, offering words of support and a friendly pat on the back. By the end of the visit, it was dark out. Our office is not in a great part of town, so I walked her out to her car. We ended up going to Starbucks together. By the end of the evening, we had agreed to meet for coffee again the next day after work.

When I look back now, I clearly see all the red flags, but at the time, each step was so trifling, I completely missed how things were escalating."

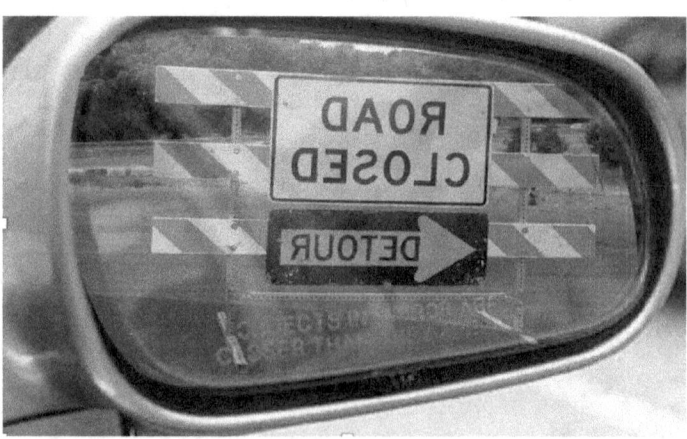

Warning signs are not always easy to spot, especially when you're preoccupied. Some, like the clinician's initial attraction to Beth in the story, are vague feelings, quickly swallowed up in the activities of the moment. Others are easily dismissed as inconsequential or missed entirely in the rush to care for someone in distress.

All too often, as in the preceding story, the signs of approaching danger only become obvious as we look back on what's happened—like a road sign noticed too late in the rearview mirror.

Red-Flag Moments

In an ideal world, we would all have the insight, and the time, to realize what we are feeling at every moment and why. In the real world of back-to-back appointments, it's more reasonable to familiarize yourself with common warning signs—red-flag moments—that can alert you to potential danger even when you are otherwise preoccupied.

Like the bumpy "rumble strips" edging highways, warning signs can jolt you into awareness of potential danger, but only if you are sensitized to them. If the clinician in the story had known ahead of time the significance and value of red-flag moments, each of the following warning signs would have caught his attention and helped him slow down and change course.

- <u>Doing something you don't ordinarily do</u> — like communicating with patients on social media, extending the time of office visits...

- <u>Socializing with patients</u> — even in the parking lot or a coffee shop...

- <u>Touching a patient without permission</u> — a sympathetic pat, a congratulatory hug...

Consider the following warning signs (in addition to the three above). Each is a symptom of potential problems and should be considered as carefully as any physical symptom. Just as a rapid pulse prompts you to consider possible medical issues, each warning sign should prompt you to consider potential boundary violations.

- <u>Accepting gifts from a patient</u> — It's gratifying to know you are appreciated, and some clinicians are comfortable accepting small token gifts, but if the situation makes you feel awkward, stop and ask yourself if the patient might be looking for something in return—possibly preferential treatment or a personal relationship? If the gift is valuable, it can easily be perceived as a tip or a bribe. That may not be what the patient intends, but remember the second law of professional boundaries: If it looks bad, it is bad.

  It's a good idea to establish an office policy about what gifts are and are not acceptable, and how to handle awkward situations (some gifts might be shared with staff or donated to a charity, for instance).

- <u>Lending money to a patient</u> — The moment you provide personal help to a patient, no matter how well intended, you are creating a dual relationship. Your patient may be embarrassed by your generosity or even resent it. They may avoid appointments until they have repaid the loan, or feel they need to reciprocate, creating even more confusion of roles.

- <u>Waiving or reducing your standard fee</u> — Whenever you are tempted to reduce your fee or waive it entirely, stop and consider how it might be perceived by others, especially insurance providers. It is illegal to charge less than Medicare would pay for a given service or procedure. You can make exceptions for someone who is financially needy, but you must document that you have done your best to verify their need. Waiving a co-pay for dental treatment in Canada is insurance fraud and could lead to fines or loss of license for the dentist. Again, it's best to have an established office policy that follows the law, perhaps with a sliding scale based on some documented evidence of hardship if legally permissible.

- <u>Inappropriately sharing information or problems with patients</u> — Briefly sharing a personal experience related to a patient's care is reasonable ("I had a similar injury, so I understand how painful it is.") But if you find yourself confiding in a patient or sharing personal information more generally, you are undermining the clinician-patient relationship by reversing roles. The patient is now focusing on your problems, instead of the other way around. The same is true when you share office gossip or complain about a colleague. Whenever you find yourself sharing more than is helpful to the patient, stop and think.

- <u>Saying or doing anything that could reasonably be interpreted as flirting</u> — Some patients are habitually flirtatious. Others may enjoy the sense of power they gain by flirting or may genuinely be attracted to you. It doesn't matter. It is never a good idea to reciprocate, even in a joking or playful way. Any time you are tempted to flirt, regardless of who started it, take it as a warning sign and consider where you are headed.

- <u>Showing favoritism</u> — It is natural to care about some patients more than others, often because they remind you of someone else or some other situation in your life. But the moment you start to do more for these patients, you are essentially short-changing all your other patients. A good rule of thumb is to never do anything for one patient you wouldn't want other patients to find out about, whether it's seeing them after hours or sharing financial advice. And any time you realize you are favoring one patient over others, stop and think about why—

before someone else asks you.

- <u>Believing you are the only one who can help a patient</u> — The moment you begin thinking no one else can do what you can for a patient, alarm bells should go off in your head. You may be responding to a personal need to be seen as heroic. You may have become so personally invested in the patient, you aren't willing to "share" them with anyone else. Whatever the reason, the more intensely you want to be the one and only, the more you should stop and consider what's really going on.

Dr. Elliot had been treating Edna, an elderly woman, for years, and was both concerned and saddened to see her health deteriorating. When he realized she, too, was becoming anxious about her increasing frailty, he suggested she might want to consult with a therapist. But Edna didn't like the idea of talking to a "stranger"

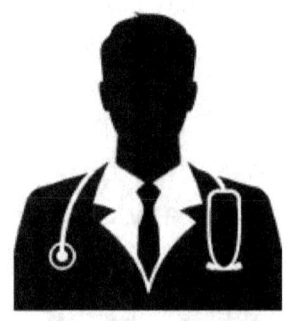

and asked if Dr. Elliot could help her himself. He knew he probably should not, but the physician could not stand the idea of Edna living alone in emotional pain. Believing he was the only one she would trust to care for her, he began seeing her on a regular basis and prescribing antidepressants.

Case File *After a few months, Edna's daughter came to visit and found her mother seriously depressed. She urged her mother to see a psychiatrist, but Edna assured her that Dr. Elliot was taking care of her, and didn't want to offend him by seeing anyone else. The daughter was outraged that the internist had been providing psychiatric care and complained to the state board.*

The board charged Dr. Elliot with practicing outside

his scope of practice. His license was suspended for a year.

Clusters Of Concern

Red-flag moments take on added significance when they become part of a pattern. The most common pattern, of course, is the slippery slope itself, a series of increasingly severe incidents. But thoughts and behavior that cluster around a common core are equally concerning. Just as the individual pixels in a digital image seem meaningless until you step back and see the whole, so can seemingly idle musings and innocuous actions paint a disturbing picture when you get some distance and view them together.

Hugging patients is far more concerning if you also tell patients off-color jokes and comment on their appearance. In such a case, it's not the increasing severity of your actions that heightens concern, but the clustering of related incidents.

Patterns like these are often difficult to detect. We're much better at spotting other people's problems than we are at noticing our own. That's why it's a good idea to enlist others' help in spotting potential problems.

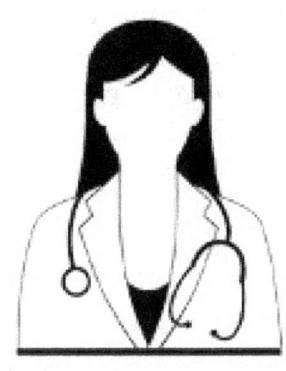

When Dr. Vincent, a new hire in a thriving practice, told the senior partner, Dr. Aldrich, about a great business deal a patient had mentioned, Dr. Aldrich expressed concern. She cautioned Dr. Vincent against entering any kind of business relationship with a patient.

A few weeks later, one of the nurses told Dr. Aldrich that Dr. Vincent had started referring patients specifically to a new lab in town. When Dr. Aldrich asked her col-

league why she was using the lab, she blushed and said the lab belonged to a good friend and she was trying to help him get off to a good start. Dr. Aldrich told the younger physician she was starting to see a troubling pattern. First there was the interest in a business deal with a patient and now she was once again allowing personal business concerns to affect patient care.

Dr. Vincent protested that she would never compromise the welfare of her patients and that her patients had told her they preferred the new lab to the old one. But when Dr. Vincent mentioned the discussion to her husband, he reminded her about her upcoming trip to a medical conference in the Bahamas. Did not the invitation come from a drug rep hoping to increase business from the practice?

Dr. Vincent not only turned down the trip, she thanked Dr. Aldrich for alerting her to the pattern she was seeing. They agreed that they would meet once a month for a while to review any similar issues that might come up.

Inattentional blindness[19]

It's surprisingly easy to miss warning signs that seem obvious in hindsight, especially when you're focused on other concerns. "When people devote their attention to a particular area or aspect of their visual world, they tend not to notice unexpected objects, even when those unexpected objects are salient, potentially important, and appear right where they are looking," write psychologists Daniel Simons and Christopher Chabris in their best-selling book, *The Invisible Gorilla*.[20]

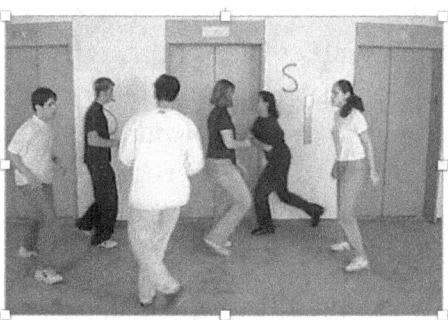

Video 1: Selective Attention Test
https://youtu.be/vJG698U2Mvo

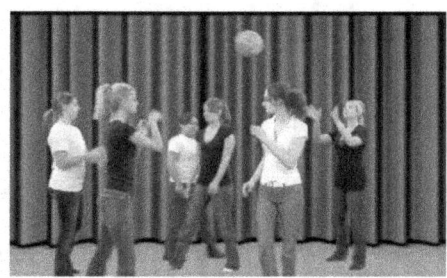

Video 2: The Monkey Business Illusion
https://youtu.be/IGQmdoK_ZfY

The title refers to a video of theirs that has been viewed online more than 16 million times. Before the video begins, viewers are challenged to count how many times people in the video pass a basketball to each other. Focused on this task, about 50% of those watching fail to notice that a person in a gorilla suit walks into the middle of the game, thumps its chest and walks off. If you find such inattentional blindness hard to believe, try watching Video 1: Selective Attention Test on the following page.

Of course, now that you know about the gorilla, you will probably be able to spot it as you count the basketball passes, just as you are more likely to spot red flags in your practice when you are actively thinking about them. But watch Video 2: The Monkey Business Illusion and see for yourself how susceptible you are to inattentional blindness, even when you know what to expect.

These light hearted gorilla videos highlight how easy it is to miss red flags like those listed above as you focus intently on your work. As the videos make abundantly clear, unless you make a conscious effort to stay alert to potential boundary violations, chances are very good that you will miss problems that are right in front of you.

The Value Of A Good Scare

If the violation is relatively minor, regulators will sometimes let first offenders off with a warning or a few months of probation. All too often, the offender breathes a sigh of relief and goes back to business as usual. That is a serious mistake for two reasons.

First, minor offenses are warning signs. In most cases, they indicate a potentially serious problem. A minor bookkeeping problem is probably a sign of weak oversight or poorly trained staff. A chiropractor who manages to explain away a misunderstood joke is very likely telling jokes and making remarks too casually for her own good. Someone who ignores a mild board or college action is throwing away a rare opportunity to make changes before it's too late.

Second, no matter how minor, a first offense is a magnifier. You may forget about it; the board or college will not. If another complaint is filed against you, you will appear before your regulator as a repeat offender. And you can expect a far less understanding reception.

> *When Dr. Oppenheimer, a psychologist, hugged her patient, George, at his mother's funeral, she meant only to be supportive. He thought otherwise and hugged her back with other intentions. When Dr. Oppenheimer protested, George became angry and defensive and accused her of inappropriately touching him.*

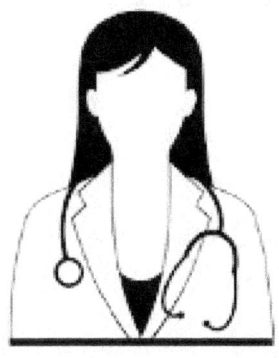

Case File

Fortunately for Dr. Oppenheimer, others at the funeral were willing to corroborate her version of events and her regulator let her off with a warning. But a year later, she was charged again, this time for hugging a teenage patient. Unable to handle the unfamiliar feelings the hug elicited, the young man rushed out and told his parents the psychologist had "come on to" him.

When she appeared before her regulator this time, they saw a pattern. She was guilty of at least poor judgment, at worst sexual exploitation of her patients. Dr. Oppenheimer's license was suspended for a year and she remained on probation for a year after that.

Takeaways

- Minor mistakes can easily lead to serious consequences.
- As the clinician, you are responsible for managing cultural conflicts with patients.
- Social media, email, and texting all pose significant challenges.
- Focused on patient satisfaction, some hospitals inadvertently foster unprofessional behavior.

  Regardless, it is the clinician who is held responsible by the patient and the board/college.
- One of the most common problems with EHR systems is the auto-populate feature.
- The Entitled Clinician: With experience and age comes an impatience with rules and regulations.

- The Distant Clinician: By viewing patients in pain as mere cases to be solved, the Distant Physician gains control.

- The Familiar Clinician: The failure to take charge is essentially a refusal to set limits.

- To maintain professional boundaries, clinicians must cultivate a full personal life and identity outside of work.

- Unacknowledged personal issues can overwhelm rational analysis and self-control. *Coming to terms with them is one of the most important things you can do to protect yourself.*

- Red-flag moments can alert you to potential danger, even when you are otherwise preoccupied.

- Red-flag moments take on added significance when they become part of a pattern.

- Minor offenses are warning signs. In most cases, they indicate a potentially serious problem.

The Four Laws of Professional Boundaries

Everyone has a violation potential which is constantly changing.

Perception is 9/10 of the law.

Protect yourself at all times.

The board (or college) decides what's right, not you.

PART 3:
Mastering the Basics

Critical Moments in Your Career o Best Practices

The challenges you face vary throughout your career, and so does your violation potential, or VP. Many factors influence your VP, including your level of experience, professional status, personal relationships, age, and health, among many others. Profound loss and great joy, tedium, and triumph —all are challenging. No two people are exactly alike, of course, but there are certain moments in life when your VP is likely to soar.

Critical Moments in Your Career

Seniority

The most commonly expressed concern about older clinicians is how the aging process can affect their care of patients. But it's not just mental acuity and physical stamina that raise senior clinicians' VP; it's ethical complacency. After decades of practice, many believe their spotless record is a testament to their innate goodness. Convinced that their own moral rectitude has stood the test of time, they relax their vigilance. Others with less experience may need to pay close attention to the rules and regulations; they themselves are beyond that, or so they imagine.

It's this sense of invulnerability that trips up experienced clinicians. They start taking a more relaxed approach to patient visits, dismissing complaints as par for the course. They become overbearing and condescending with staff and younger colleagues, angrily rejecting well-meaning and often important observations and suggestions. Warnings from administrators and colleagues are brushed aside, until eventually, a regulator takes disciplinary action.

Training

Professional students and young clinicians face the opposite challenge. Lack of experience and confidence often lead them to make poor judgments when confronted with a boundary challenge. Among the most common boundary issues for medical trainees:

- Thinking like a student, not a professional: Concerns about grades, graduation and residency placement make students especially vulnerable to fraud violations, including: falsifying patient logs, plagiarism, lying or deception, cheating on tests, and exaggerating accomplishments on applications.

- Acting like a pal, instead of a professional: Uncomfortable with authority and eager to help, students sometimes give patients money for prescriptions, offer them rides home, or tell them to call their personal cell phone number if they have a question.

- Accepting gifts: Refusing gifts from a grateful patient can seem rude, but failing to do so can create a risky sense of obligation. A patient who has given you something of value is all too likely to expect something of equal value in return. According to the Texas Medical Association, "It is particularly dangerous in the case of a student, who may feel obligated to provide "special care" in the form of sexual favors or other inappropriate gestures because the student cannot realistically provide medical care."

- Prescribing for family and friends: A resident may relish the feeling of importance they get when writing a prescription for a family member or friend, or they may find it difficult to refuse helping someone they are close to. Yet even when the activity isn't explicitly prohibited, casual prescribing is always a violation if it is done, as is almost always the case, without examining the person first or updating their medical records afterwards.

- Becoming romantically or sexually involved with someone in your care: Without proper training, naïve students and residents can find it hard to accept that there is no such thing as a consensual relationship with someone who is dependent on you. A resident may invite a student they are supervising out for a drink; a student may flirt with a patient in their care. The problem, of course, is that the power differential—between caregiver and patient or between resident and student—makes such overtures inherently coercive.

Retirement

Many clinicians resist retiring. The profession has been so

central to their lives and so integral to their sense of self-worth that the thought of letting go is simply too threatening to contemplate. "For most of us, the practice isn't a job: It's more of a calling," said Glen Gabbard, MD. A clinical professor of psychiatry at Baylor College of Medicine and an expert in physician health and professionalism, Gabbard was speaking at an AMA session on retirement. "One of the things that's unique about physicians is that who we are— our identity—is so wrapped up in being a physician."[21]

Even those who do let go and retire often keep a tight grip on their license and prescription pad—which is how they run afoul of professional boundaries. No longer in practice, these licensed retirees generally fail to keep up with the latest developments. Still, they cannot resist offering medical advice and prescribing for family and friends, almost always without taking adequate histories and updating patients' charts.

Boards are quick to discipline such lax professional behavior, and physicians who have retired after a long and distinguished career may end up with a tarnished reputation, not to mention other penalties.

Mental Illness

According to the 2018 Medscape National Report on Physician Burnout and Depression, nearly two-thirds of U.S. physicians say they feel burned out (42%), depressed (15%) or both (14%).[22] Yet fully two-thirds of those who reported burnout and depression on the Medscape survey said they were not seeking professional help and never had.

While clinicians regularly advise patients struggling with mental health issues to seek professional help, they themselves are taught to tough it out in silence. "They learn early in their training to hold the line, to come across as stoic, to turn up ready for work come what may, and never to admit to their vulnerabilities," says Dr. Clare Gerada, medical director of England's Practitioner Health Programme and a former chair of the Royal College of General Practitioners.[23]

Worse, medical boards have sidelined physicians who admit seeking mental health help and disciplined others for hiding the fact. Caught in this catch-22, many physicians ask colleagues to provide "hallway prescriptions" or try to medicate themselves, sometimes with anti-depressants but all too often with alcohol or opioids.

Recent efforts suggest boards and colleges are rethinking their policies. For example, the CMPA, in its role to help manage risk and contribute to safe medical care, urges regulatory colleges to collect only that information that might impact a physician's ability to practice, rather than to collect information about conditions a physician has ever had in their life (see https://www.cmpa-acpm.ca/en/advice-publications/browse-articles/2012/a-medico-legal-perspective-on-physician-health-and-wellness-removing-barriers-to-treatment-of-physician-patients). However, the culture of medicine is likely to evolve slowly. In the meantime, it's important to recognize that when it comes to protecting your career and your patients, your mental health is every bit as important as your physical health.

Family And Financial Stress

You are already well aware of how stressful your professional life is and how difficult it can be to maintain a healthy work-life balance. When your personal life is also stressful, the risk of making a mistake and crossing a boundary intensifies dramatically. Family issues are the most obvious and common source of stress. Marital problems, aging parents, rebellious teenagers—all of these personal issues can raise your violation potential. In recent years, financial pressures have increased as well.

As the cost of becoming a doctor has skyrocketed, so has the level of financial insecurity. Tuition for private medical schools has nearly tripled over the past 30 years and public medical school tuition has grown even faster. As a result, the average student debt at graduation is now $166,750. And this mountain of debt generally continues to grow over the ensuing years of low-paying residency and fellowships. According to James M. Dahle, author of *The White Coat Investor: A Doctor's Guide To Personal Finance And Investing*, "This debt load, when coupled with the traditionally poor financial management habits of physicians and a financial services industry that has traditionally targeted doctors as "whales" to be harpooned, is causing severe financial difficulties for a rapidly rising percentage of physicians."[24]

But educational debt, practice start-up costs, and other family matters create financial pressures on all clinicians. Even when healthcare professionals eventually crawl out from under their student debt or other financial obligations, they often feel pressure to make up for lost time—and all too often end up on the wrong side of a professional boundary.

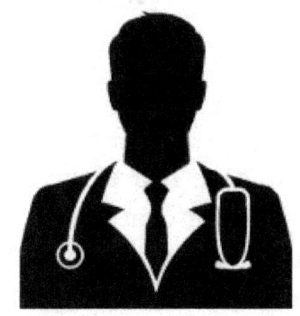
Case File

Dr. Krebs was elated. Newly married, with a booming practice, he had purchased a large house in the suburbs. It was more than he could afford at the moment, but he felt certain his finances would strengthen as his business grew.

Soon after closing on the house, however, a large practice opened down the street and Dr. Krebs began losing patients. The variable rate mortgage on the house was growing increasingly burdensome and his wife needed surgery.

As his financial situation worsened, Dr. Krebs began asking colleagues for referrals. A surgeon at the hospital mentioned a patient recovering from a mastectomy who might benefit from Dr. Krebs 'care after she was discharged. WIth unpaid bills piling up, Dr. Krebs went ahead and examined the patient while she was still in the hospital, explaining that the surgeon had asked for a consult.

When the woman mentioned the examination, she was alarmed to learn that her surgeon had not asked Dr. Krebs to see her. Feeling violated, she complained to the hospital and the medical board. Since neither the patient nor the surgeon had sanctioned the intimate examination, Dr.
Krebs was arrested for sexual assault. While the criminal charges were ultimately reduced, the board revoked his license.

Midlife

When you're a young adult just starting out, you feel you can do anything. By the time you've cleared most of life's hurdles, you're satisfied with what you've done. It's the middle, when you're in your prime but nearing the top of the career ladder, that you're most likely to feel dissatisfied. Research shows that for most of us, life follows a U-shaped curve, with highs at either end and a valley of discontent in midlife.

Clinicians are as likely as anyone else to suffer doubts and frustrations as they enter this period, maybe more so. The everyday demands of modern health care are draining enough. Frustrated by mounting responsibilities and diminishing opportunities, middle-aged physicians, nurses and other clinicians often feel less inspired by medicine than trapped. For them, the very idea of breaking the rules takes on a new luster and making bold, if rash decisions seems exhilarating. There are plenty of benefits to midlife reassessment, but it's also a time to realize you are apt to do something you will later regret.

Best Practices

It's important for patients to develop good health habits, regardless of their particular ailments. The same is true for good work-life habits for clinicians. The best practices described below will help you strengthen your practice and protect your career no matter what particular issues are troubling you. Instituting these good habits won't guarantee a trouble-free future any more than eating a healthy diet and exercising regularly guarantees a lifetime of good health. But ignoring them is asking for trouble.

Care For Yourself

You devote your life to caring for others, but probably neglect caring for yourself. This is neither noble nor smart. Your ability to meet your patients' needs is totally dependent on your own physical and mental health.

- At a minimum, you should have a regular primary care provider and work with them to maintain your physical wellbeing. This should be too obvious to need saying, but the number of clinicians who neglect such rudimentary self-care is distressingly high.

- You also, of course, need to attend to your emotional health. You may think that seeking help from mental health professionals will damage your career, but denying emotional pain only intensifies suffering and refusing treatment endangers both your career and your patients—not to mention family and friends. Most US states, all Canadian provinces, and two of the territories (not the Northwest Territory) have physician health programs that provide assessment and assistance to physicians with mental and emotional issues and impairment. Similarly, the other clinical professions offer professional health programs, often as part of a regulatory college or a state or province's professional association (e.g., College of Nurses of Ontario Nurses' Health Program, Michigan Health Professional Recovery Program).

Take Time For Yourself

Regardless of how well you tend to your physical and mental health, you are headed for serious trouble if you are one of the many clinicians who mistakenly believe their professional lives make it impossible to have any significant personal life. Balancing your personal and professional lives is not a zero-sum game. The time you spend away from work allows you to recharge your batteries and return to work emotionally equipped to care for others. The time you spend at work gives you the space you need to see personal challenges from a new perspective.

Perhaps most importantly, when you find intimacy and companionship with friends and family, you no longer crave them at work. The only way to avoid or escape the "role vacuum" described by Peter Graham is to maintain a robust and fulfilling personal life.

"Part of being a doctor involves protecting yourself," notes Graham. "It involves setting boundaries so that you have time to have a private life, where you can have a differentiated self." It's only by having a range of different experiences — as a doctor, a parent, a child, a friend and a neighbor, for instance—that you can access different perspectives.

"Part of what we teach people is that you have to live your life in such a way that maintaining that two-part perspective is possible," explains Graham. "If the only experience you have when you're awake is working with patients, dealing with suffering, and you don't have time and the opportunity to have alternative experiences, then all that's left is constant immersion. The doctor who's always on call has no chance to experience a different perspective on the world."[25]

Well-maintained boundaries also allow clinicians to take crucial time for themselves, so they can recharge their batteries. It takes a good deal of emotional strength to hold on to your own perspective while listening to and empathizing with patient after patient. "That's why it's so important for physicians to get away from work and rejuvenate themselves," says Graham, "to take the time to think and talk to other people about the reality of what they are going through."

Most importantly, when you find intimacy and companionship with friends and family, you no longer crave them at work.

Don't Use Work As An Escape

Clinicians are not the only ones who turn to work for solace and escape, but the consequences for them and their patients are far more serious. When you use your practice to avoid personal pain, you are putting your own needs ahead of your patients'—a fundamental violation of your fiduciary responsibility. And the transient ease you find does nothing to solve the underlying problem, which worsens, causing even more problems.

> *Gail Hirsch, a nurse-midwife, had gotten through a rocky time by immersing herself in her work. She had refused to take time off when her mother passed away unexpectedly, and continued working long hours after learning that her teenage son was addicted to drugs. Her husband complained that she was neglecting her family and now*

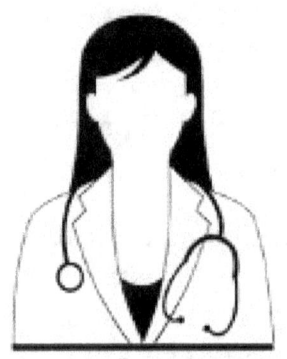

Case File

she was worried about her marriage.

Unable to sleep, she asked a colleague for a prescription. When he refused to renew it, she began self-medicating with alcohol and drug samples meant for patients. When her supervisor reprimanded her for sloppy work, she reacted angrily and stormed out of the office, berating a member of the staff on the way out.

The board cited her for unprofessional conduct, suspended her license for six months, and told her it would not consider reinstating it until she had satisfactorily completed remedial classes and gone for counseling.

Care For Others, But Not Too Much

Clinicians who fail to empathize with patients while taking a history or conducting a physical examination can come across as callous or even aggressive. Others who suppress empathy can lose a sense of purpose and end up feeling dehumanized. Yet caring too much can be just as damaging. Clinicians who suffer from "pathological empathy" get tangled up in the emotional web generated by their patients and lose objectivity. In extreme cases, such clinicians identify so closely with a patient that they end up in a kind of dual relationship, relating to the patient both as a separate person and as a proxy for themselves.

According to Graham, the key to resolving this conflict is learning to develop a higher-order empathy. "Empathy involves two levels," he explains, "being able to imagine the subjective emotional experience of another person from their perspective, while simultaneously being able to maintain your own separate feelings and perspective." When dealing with a patient who is "exuding this affect and these feelings," says Graham, the clinician has to "accurately identify with that, understand where it's coming from, but at the same time maintain a professional perspective with the specific intention of a clinician, which is to care for the patient."

"Every school of thought in psychology and psychiatry has their own language for this mental position," notes Graham. Some psychoanalytically oriented researchers use the term "mentalization," while others talk about "emotional intelligence" or "reflective functioning." Each of these approaches is distinct, but all highlight the desirability of emotionally understanding both what someone else is feeling and what you yourself are feeling, and the importance of maintaining a clear separation between the two.

As difficult as it is to achieve this dual awareness, the fact is that people have been doing it for thousands of years. Buddhist monks are able to care about and care for others, emotionally connect with people in pain, and maintain the distance needed to help relieve their pain. Tania Singer, professor of Neuroscience and Neuroeconomics at the University of Zurich, conducted brain scans of both Buddhist monks and non-meditators as they watched videos of people suffering. According to an article in *Wired*, the fMRI scans of the monks' brains "showed heightened activity in areas that are important to care, nurturing and positive social affiliation. In non-meditators, the videos were more likely to trigger the brain areas associated with unpleasant feelings of sadness and pain."[26]

This ability to emotionally understand what another is feeling, while at the same time focusing on ways to help, has roots even deeper than the Buddhist tradition. One monk compared what he felt while watching the videos to "the warm, loving, caring feeling" that a mother feels towards a crying child—the ability to feel a strong emotional connection and maintain the distance needed to provide care.

Equitable Care Demands Cultural Sensitivity

The ability to care for patients from different backgrounds grows more critical every day. Numerous studies have shown that large minority segments of both the U.S. and Canadian populations are receiving substandard care. The problem is less outright prejudice than a lack of cultural sensitivity. The same words and behavior can mean very different things depending on your patient's background. You may assume someone is feeling embarrassed or guilty if they avoid looking you in the eye, but in much of the world avoiding eye contact is a show of respect.

And cultural differences are not limited by geography. Religion, ethnicity, sexual orientation and social class all influence the assumptions we make and the way we behave. That applies to your patients and to you, too. If you have a patient from a background different from yours, it's important to follow some basic guidelines[27]:

- **Don't make assumptions.** Patients from other parts of the world might not be familiar with certain types of diseases seen in the US or Canada. Breast cancer, for instance, is practically unknown in parts of Africa, the Middle East, and Asia.

- **Explain every detail.** Patients whose native language is not English may have a difficult time understanding medical jargon.

- **Ask about alternative approaches to healing.** Many cultures may use herbal remedies or other alternative treatments that could have a potentially harmful interaction with Western medicine.

- **Withhold judgments.** Some cultures place high

value on extended family members, who may fill a patient's room, or interdependence instead of independence when it comes to self-care routines such as bathing and eating.

Reduce the risk of "he said, she said" incidents

- **Good medical records are your first line of defense** when regulators, patients, insurance companies, or hospitals question your performance or accuse you of a violation. If a patient complains that you said or did something inappropriate, it is not enough to simply deny it. You are in a much better position if you have a contemporaneous medical record that documents your version of events.

    The cardinal rule is simple: If you don't write it down, it didn't happen. Remember the case cited earlier about the patient who patted her doctor on the butt. Feeling embarrassed and rejected when Dr. Greely asked her to stop, the patient tried to deflect her guilt by complaining that the physician had patted *her* on the butt. A note in the medical record would have confirmed the doctor's version, but he didn't write anything down and ended up being disciplined by the board.

- **Medical chaperones are like malpractice insurance—they protect you from danger you hope never to encounter.** Most states now require US physicians to carry malpractice insurance—as Canadian physicians in private practice or hospitals are required—even if you've gone 20 years without an issue. The likelihood of your being sued may be small, but the potential consequences are huge. The same holds true for boundary violations. No matter how confident you are that you will never violate a boundary, seeing patients without a chaperone exposes you to an unacceptable level of risk.

Having a chaperone to back you up does not guarantee safety, but it comes close. In the vast majority of cases, when a clinician has a chaperone, any complaints that are filed are quickly resolved in the clinician's favor. Cases in which there is no chaperone generally stretch on for months and the final judgment is far less predictable.

Today, the American Medical Association's Code of Ethics, the American College of Obstetrics and Gynecology, the American Academy of Pediatrics, the American College of Physicians, and several Canadian regulatory colleges all recommend the use of chaperones, at least in certain situations. Since misperception and miscommunication can happen at any time with any patient, it's best to use a chaperone every time you are with a patient, not just during intimate exams. In fact, among the cases we hear about at PBI Education, the majority of complaints about improper touching stem from non-intimate, unchaperoned cases.

If the blanket use of chaperones is impractical for you, at least be sure to have a chaperone in the room any time you conduct an intimate exam. (Most people define an intimate exam as one that involves the pelvis or female breast. However, many other types of exams could also be considered intimate, such as exams of the eyes and skin.) If you practice in Alabama, Delaware, Georgia, Montana, New Jersey, Ohio or Tennessee, you are required to do so by law even if you are not mandated through restrictions on your license (no such mandates exist in Canada). If you live outside these seven states, do it anyway. Even if you are a female gynecologist or a male urologist examining a male patient, chaperones should always be present when you are examining genitalia, buttocks or breasts. The days of making facile assumptions about sexual orientation and gender identification are gone, and you have no way of knowing who will be sensitive to what.

There will be times when patients themselves object to having a chaperone in the room. So make the practice a policy, which would include explaining the role of the chaperone and the reason the policy exists. (See the CMPA article https://www.cmpa-acpm.ca/en/advice-publications/browse-articles/2019/is-it-time-to-rethink-your-use-of-chaperones for more guidance.) If a patient still objects, make a decision about whether or not you are willing to take the risk of conducting an intimate exam without a chaperone. If you're not, explain to your patient that as a matter of policy you won't be able to examine them, document their refusal in their chart and refer them to someone else if they wish.

> **Use of Chaperones**
> **AMA Code of Medical Ethics Opinion 1.2.4**
>
> Efforts to provide a comfortable and considerate atmosphere for the patient and the physician are part of respecting patients' dignity. These efforts may include providing appropriate gowns, private facilities for undressing, sensitive use of draping, and clearly explaining various components of the physical examination. They also include having chaperones available. Having chaperones present can also help prevent misunderstandings between patient and physician.
>
> Physicians should:
>
> (a) Adopt a policy that patients are free to request a chaperone and ensure that the policy is communicated to patients.
>
> (b) Always honor a patient's request to have a chaperone.
>
> (c) Have an authorized member of the health care team serve as a chaperone. Physicians should establish clear expectations that chaperones will uphold professional standards of privacy and confidentiality.

- **Can you afford a chaperone?** The obvious answer is that you cannot afford to be without one. If you think a chaperone is expensive, consider the cost of defending yourself. An inexpensive lawyer is going to cost you at least $300 an hour, and without a chaperone, "he said, she said" cases burn up a lot of hours.

The simplest way to reduce the costs involved is to use people already on staff as chaperones. (Don't make the mistake of assuming a patient's family members can serve the purpose. They are unlikely to be objective and will rarely testify in your favor.) In a perfect world, the staff member you employ will have enough medical training to know what is appropriate during an exam and be able to help reassure nervous patients. If that's not always possible, it's better to have someone than no one. If the chaperone is not medically trained, you should prepare them ahead of time by explaining what they will be seeing and what you'll be doing, and answer any questions afterward. It's also important that they understand and respect the rules about patient confidentiality.

One caveat about asking existing staff to serve as chaperones: having worked with you and for you, they may feel uneasy about speaking up in front of a patient or even confronting you in private.

Scribes, who have been trained in specific specialties, are a good cost-saving option. Advocates claim they more than pay for themselves by increasing clinicians' efficiency and effectiveness. And since the scribe is already in the room, it costs nothing extra to have them serve as a chaperone. What's more, patients tend to prefer chaperones who are actively doing something, rather than just sitting and watching them. The downside is that the scribe's attention is divided and they are more likely to miss something than someone whose sole job is to monitor the patient's safety and comfort level.

A word of caution: In your zeal to be efficient, resist the temptation to use your chaperone as a gofer. A chaperone should stick with you like a shadow. They should not leave the room while you are with the patient and they should not stay behind if you leave the room.

Realizing the young woman he was examining was nervous, Dr. Quentin, a breast surgeon, made sure to have a chaperone in the room during the exam. He was shocked when he was notified soon after that the patient had complained to the hospital's Patient Liaison Officer, claiming that Dr. Quentin had fondled her and made suggestive

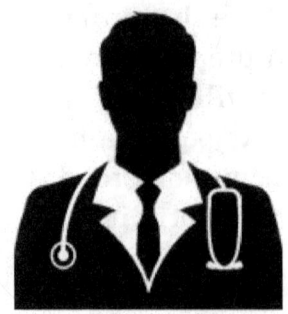

Case File

comments.

In the subsequent hearing, the chaperone testified on the surgeon's behalf. But when asked if she had left the room at any point, the chaperone recalled leaving to grab a mammogram the doctor wanted to consult. Asked how long Dr. Quentin had been alone with the patient, the chaperone estimated about eight seconds. The review committee reprimanded the surgeon and put him on probation for six months, during which time he was required to have a chaperone with him at all times.

Maintain Professional-Quality Records

Few aspects of medicine are more basic than record keeping, or more misunderstood. Clinicians generally learn that records have to be legible, contemporaneous, and complete. The legible part is clear enough. Contemporaneous is a relative term. Most regulators agree it means as soon as possible after the patient was seen. Again, given the rarity of perfect recall, it's clear why it's a mistake to wait too long, or see too many other patients, before writing up notes.

- **Keep *complete* records.** But when it comes to keeping "complete records," many clinicians fail to grasp what's involved. Today, boards and colleges insist that a record "stand on its own." That means that when the next provider looks at that record, they have to be able to understand from start to finish what's been done and why. The record should include a good sense of the relevant history up to that point, as well as medical justifications for all the clinical decisions a provider makes.

In the past, you could think of a patient's whole medical record as a novel. If you read just the notes from one visit, it would be like reading a single chapter in the middle of the book: you might not understand who all the characters were or every aspect of the plot. Well now, regulators want each individual record to be a short story, with a beginning, middle and end—complete and intelligible all on its own.

- **Document functionality.** If a patient's hypertension is being successfully treated by medication, it is not enough to simply renew the prescription and add a quick note. You must document the fact that that the patient's blood pressure is within acceptable limits under the medication. Given today's rampant opioid epidemic, it is especially important that you fully document the extent to which a patient's functionality is improved by the prescription of a controlled substance.
- **Beware of the auto-populate feature in electronic health records.** A lot has been written about the pros and cons of electronic health records. One of the pros is supposed to be the time saved when the software automatically populates certain information. But this auto-populate feature has to be carefully monitored. Providers run into problems when they fail to double check that all of the auto-populated fields contain correct data.
- **Good record keeping includes good bookkeeping**. According to the Department of Health and Human Services (HHS), "When you submit a claim for services performed for a Medicare patient, you are filing a bill with the Federal Government and certifying you earned the payment requested and complied with the billing requirements. If you knew *or should have known* the submitted claim was false, then the attempt to

collect payment constitutes a violation."[28]

Improper coding, especially up-coding, is a federal crime, as is billing for something already covered by a global fee (billing for an evaluation and management service the day after surgery, for instance). Signing off on a subordinate's actions without first reviewing them is also a federal offense if the insurance provider is Medicare or Medicaid. The extent of fraud in Canada may be more difficult to detect and investigate than in the U.S. because there is no federal oversight for this problem, according to an article in the Canadian Medical Association Journal (https://www.ncbi.nlm.nih.gov/pmc/articles/PMC3537805/).
And in contrast with the U.S., Canadian health ministries typically regard inaccurate billings as mistakes rather than fraud, and require physicians to pay back the excess funds they were paid.

Documentation is key. If Medicare suspects a problem, its investigators will examine your clinical records as well as your books. If the two don't jibe, or if your documentation does not support the claims you submit, you are in violation of federal law and subject to criminal prosecution. Similarly, if there is a mismatch between documentation and billings, the provincial Ministry of Health will initiate an investigation that could lead to repayment of excess funds and potential disciplinary action from your regulatory college.

Beware Of Conflicts Of Interest

Any time your own self-interest—whether it's making money, advancing your career or simply satisfying your scientific curiosity—clouds your focus on what's best for your patient, you have a conflict of interest. It doesn't matter if the interest actually biases your professional judgment (and making that determination is always problematic) or harms the patient in any way. The risk that it might is what defines a conflict of interest.

Of course, some conflicts of interest are more severe than others. The more likely it is to influence your judgment and the more potential for patient harm, the greater the severity. The U.S. Federal Government warns providers filing claims with Medicare of two specific conflicts of interest. These specific examples serve as good rules of thumb for any U.S. or Canadian clinician.

<u>Relationships with other providers:</u> You are likely to encounter numerous temptations to align yourself with others in health care. Whether the other party is a lab, a clinic, a specialist or a hospital, be wary. Is the offer better than you would expect it to be? Are you being asked to make referrals as part of the deal? Whether or not referrals are explicitly mentioned, are you more likely to refer patients because of your involvement?

<u>Relationships with the pharmaceutical and medical device industries:</u> Offers from such companies can be both lucrative and prestigious, and there is no harm in accepting an offer, provided there is a legitimate link between the services you can provide and the compensation you are promised. If the company is paying for anything other than your special expertise, accepting the offer, no matter how tempting, is never a good idea.

The safest and best course of action is to be open about any conflicts that you think may bias you, or that might concern your patient. If you recommend a certain lab, refer a patient to a particular clinic, or suggest a particular procedure, clarify whether or not you stand to benefit in any way. You cannot eliminate all conflicts of interest, but telling your patient about any of potential consequence will reduce the likelihood that you will be influenced, help maintain the patient's trust, and allow the patient to make their own informed decisions.

Legally, you are obliged to follow specific rules about conflicts of interest if you accept funding from foundations, state governments, universities and the National Institutes of Health (NIH). Most regulatory colleges post guidelines pertaining to conflicts of interest on their websites. "If you are uncertain whether a conflict exists, apply the "newspaper test" and ask yourself whether you would want the arrangement to appear on the front page of your local newspaper," advises HHS.

Once A Patient, Always A Patient

When it comes to dating a former patient, the rules are dangerously ambiguous. The AMA categorically rules out romantic or sexual relationships between physicians and current patients, but offers only a vague warning about ex-patients. "Sexual or romantic relationships with former patients are unethical if the physician uses or exploits trust, knowledge, emotions, or influence derived from the previous professional relationship, or if a romantic relationship would otherwise foreseeably harm the individual."[29]

The American Psychiatric Association is more definitive, presumably because of the intense emotional interaction between psychiatrists and patients. Members are strictly prohibited from relationships with current or former patients. And the American Psychological Association's Ethics Code falls in between the other two professional associations. It prohibits members from intimate relationships with patients "for at least two years after cessation or termination of therapy," and cautions members that even after two years, they still "bear the burden of demonstrating that there has been no exploitation, in light of all relevant factors."[30] Professional codes of ethics dictate the restrictions on intimate relationships with patients or former patients, supported by the Regulated Health Professions Act in each province. For example, the College of Nurses of Ontario Code of Conduct states that "Nurses do not engage in any sexual relationship with patients while caring for them. This legislation stays in effect for one year after the end of the nurse-patient relationship." (See https://www.cno.org/globalassets/docs/prac/49040_code-of-conduct.pdf.)

Problems arise when relationships sour. That's when former patients are apt to bring charges against the clinician, even if they initiated the involvement. As always, boards and colleges consider such charges in terms of the patient's safety, not the licensee's career.

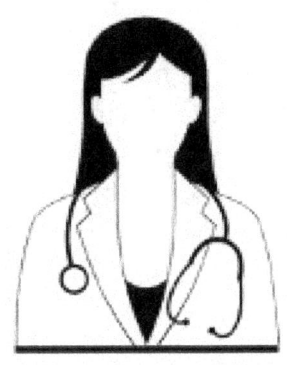
Case File

Dr. Lee, an experienced therapist, had not seen Greg, a former patient, for more than three years. After a chance meeting, they struck up a personal friendship, which gradually evolved into an intimate, but non-exclusive relationship. Or so Dr. Lee thought.

When Greg found out she was also dating other men, he became incensed and threatened his former therapist. Alarmed, Dr. Lee obtained a restraining order. The emotional toll pushed Greg back into therapy with another therapist, who after hearing his story, filed charges. Dr. Lee's license was suspended for two years.

Follow Social Media Guidelines

Online violations of all sorts are fast outstripping the ability of laws and regulations to contain them. As far back as 2010, 92% of U.S. state medical board directors reported violations of online professionalism in their jurisdiction. And according to the Federation of State Medical Boards, 71% of state boards held formal disciplinary proceedings as a result of those infractions.[31]

So the next time you pull out your laptop or reach for your phone, keep in mind the following:

- **Never say anything online that you wouldn't want a patient or colleague to hear.** One of the most common dangers people face online is that they tend to lose the inhibitions that normally keep them safe. Remember, when you say something online, it's public.

- **It's never ok to talk about patients in an unsecured environment.** A chiropractor who used social media to complain about a difficult day was careful to eliminate any details that might identify the patient he mentioned. He wasn't careful enough. The patient's wife instantly realized who he was writing about and complained. Even unsecured emails and texts are dangerous, since you never know who might read them. And once it's out there—whether it's texts, emails, or social media posts—it doesn't go away; it's there forever.

- **It's all too easy to cross state lines.** It's fine to post generic health information on a website, as many providers do, but patient-specific advice is fraught with problems. For one thing, since you don't know where the recipient lives, you might end up advising someone who lives in another jurisdiction. If you're not licensed in that jurisdiction, you can be accused of practicing your profession without a license.

- **What your staff does online is your business.** If a

staff member posts a photo or comment online that violates the law, they are not the one the board or college will target; you are. You are the captain of the ship and responsible for everything that happens in your office. Numerous physicians, dentists, advance practice nurses, and others have been disciplined for improper supervision, whether the offense was committed online or in the office.

- **Relevant digital communications must be documented.** The HIPAA privacy rule gives patients the right to access and amend protected health information. So if you use texts or emails in making a clinical decision be sure to document those communications in the patient's medical record. If you don't, you are technically in non-compliance.

- **Friending a patient is not the same as being friendly.** When a clinician friends a patient on Facebook—or invites contact through any other social networking site—she is inviting that person to see her outside of her professional role, whether on vacation or at a sporting event. Such casual intimacy can start a dangerous slide down the slippery slope to an inappropriate relationship. In fact, the 2011 California case of Roy vs. the Superior Court established that physicians who share too much personal information are inviting patients to get closer "than would be professional or appropriate."[32]

- **What you say online can and will be used against you in court.** The "e" in email stands for evidence. While most of the cases involving social media are directly related to what has happened online, most of the texts and emails that show up in court are not the reason for the case but rather evidence supporting the charges that are being brought.

- **Work phones need to be protected.** According to the American Health Information Management Association (AHIMA), "Text messages may reside on a mobile device indefinitely, where the information can be exposed to unauthorized third parties due to theft, loss, or recycling of the device."[33] To guard against this threat to privacy, be sure your phone is password protected and that any patient information is stored in a separate secure file. As noted above, be sure to use HIPAA- or PIPEDA-compliant software.

- **Personal cell phones are for personal use only.** When you talk to patients on your personal phone, you risk creating a dual relationship and raising unrealistic expectations. There have been cases in which a mental health patient has filed a complaint because a therapist, who had previously responded after hours on a personal phone, was not available when the patient needed help again.

Remember The Basics

- **The whole truth and nothing but the truth.** One of the most common ethics violations is falsifying applications for licensure or renewal. Outright lying is rare, but a surprising number of clinicians have been disciplined for inaccurately filling out questionnaires for licensure, license renewal, hospital privileges, or credentialing and continuing education, among others. Online databases have made it simple for boards, regulatory colleges, hospitals, and others to run background checks, so they will know if you exaggerate or omit anything.

you leave something out, simply because it's embarrassing or seems unimportant, the omission will almost certainly come to light. And no matter how small the crime, or how long ago it was—a teenage DUI, for instance—you've falsified your application and can expect to be sanctioned.

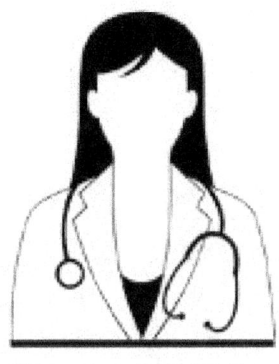

As a teenager, Christina had once been arrested for shoplifting. The judge was understanding and reduced the charge to a misdemeanor. Christina returned the dress, performed a few weeks of community service, and never again run afoul of the law.

In fact, a few years later she was the first in her family to attend college and after graduation had attended pharmacy school. When it came time to apply for her pharmacist license, she hesitated over the question asking whether she had ever been arrested. The shoplifting incident was so long ago and she had accomplished so much since then, it hardly seemed worth mentioning. Christina checked the "no" box and moved on.

The board, which routinely checked police records, quickly discovered the shoplifting arrest and denied Christina's application, citing her lack of honesty. In their letter, the board urged her to attend remedial classes on ethics before reapplying.

- **You have a duty to report.** You are far more likely to be disciplined for failing to report your own misdeeds or mistakes, but you are also ethically, and in some cases legally, obligated to report suspected violations by colleagues. Your first step should be to talk to the person about your concerns, but if they do not take the matter seriously or repeat the offense, you owe it to them, their patients, and their profession to report what you know or suspect.

- **You are the captain of the ship.** If you hire someone, whether a receptionist or practice partner, you are responsible for what they do on the job. If someone on your staff breaks patient confidentiality, harasses someone, or makes a billing error, you are the one the regulator will sanction or discipline—and the discipline can be severe.

  In one case, a physician lost his license when he signed the paperwork submitted by a physician assistant in a satellite office without first reviewing it—a clear violation of the laws governing "collaborative practices." In another, a dental surgeon ended up in jail because he failed to adequately supervise the billing company he employed. (See Part 2.)

  The greatest threat to proper supervision is allowing professional relationships with staff to collapse into personal friendships. Once again, the key is maintaining boundaries between your personal and professional lives.

- **Pay attention to current board concerns.** As you would expect, regulators tend to focus on those health care issues that loom largest at any one time. The widely publicized Larry Nassar case has drawn national attention to sexual abuse, especially of minors. Other issues may be paramount in your state, province, or territory. If Medicare fraud has been making headlines locally, it's safe to assume your state board is going to be especially vigilant in policing the rules governing reimbursements. It's a good idea to check which issues are uppermost in board members' or college members' minds by periodically scanning recent activity on their website.

<u>Currently, regulators across the U.S. and Canada are focused on the opioid epidemic.</u> If you are licensed to prescribe controlled substances, it is critically important that you understand the best practices. You'll find more information online, but here are some highlights:

- o Conduct a thorough assessment, including a detailed medical history, physical exam, baseline urine drug test and assessment of the patient's risk of opioid abuse.

- o Urine drug testing should be conducted randomly and for cause to determine if the patient is taking prescribed medication or diverting it, or taking any drugs not prescribed.

- o Use the online Prescription Monitoring Programs available in all states (except Missouri), seven provinces and Yukon Territory (not New Brunswick, Prince Edward Island, Northwest Territories, or Nunavut), to ensure that patients are not filling prescriptions from multiple providers.

- o Establish basic ground rules upfront in a signed agreement that spells out what you and the patient can expect of each other.

- o See patients on opioids every one or two months, to assess the effectiveness of the current plan and make changes as needed.

- o Keep thorough records, especially concerning functionality.

- o Given the complexities of safely tapering patients off opioids, it's best to establish upfront how this will be accomplished if needed.

Takeaways

- Your Violation Potential is likely to soar at critical times in your life.
    - Seniority: Experience breeds ethical complacency.
    - Residency: Making the transition from student to advanced trainee can be difficult.
    - Retirement: If you retire with a license, you are still subject to regulator discipline.
    - Mental illness: The health professions discourage seeking needed care.
    - Family and financial stress: Personal stress can cloud clinician's' reasoning, distort their priorities, and cause them to make poor judgments.
    - Midlife: The average age of physicians disciplined for boundary violations is 47.
- Caring for others but not yourself is neither noble nor smart.
- Balancing your personal and professional lives is not a zero-sum game. The two realms should complement each other.
- When you use work to escape personal pain, you put your own needs ahead of your patients'.
- Dual awareness is an essential—and learned—skill. You can learn to empathize with a patient's pain without losing your objectivity.
- Medical chaperones are like malpractice insurance—they protect you from danger you hope never to encounter.

- Few aspects of medicine are more basic—or more misunderstood—than record keeping.
- Any time your own self-interest clouds your focus on your patient, you have a conflict of interest.
- Once a patient always a patient.
- Violations of online professionalism are an increasingly common subject of regulator discipline.
- Check your regulator's website to learn which issues are most concerning in your area.
- Regulators in the U.S. and Canada are currently focused on the opioid epidemic.

The Four Laws of Professional Boundaries

Everyone has a violation potential which is constantly changing.

Perception is 9/10 of the law.

Protect yourself at all times.

The board (or college) decides what's right, not you.

PART 4:
Becoming a Complete Physician

Gauging Your Own Violation Potential o Putting the Formula to Work

A patient in physical pain is much more likely to seek help and follow a treatment plan than one whose illness causes little discomfort. It's the same with boundary violators. Healthcare professionals who come to a remedial course facing suspension or revocation of their license are desperate to end the emotional pain they are in. They are far more willing to confront the issues that got them into trouble and make significant changes in their lives than those who show up relatively unconcerned about the consequences of their actions.

Those who have simply had their wrists slapped—let off with a warning, say—tend to view remedial courses as a bureaucratic waste of time, like those required sexual harassment seminars you occasionally have to attend. They sit through the classes, resume their lives, and all too often end up before the board or college a second time, now as a repeat offender.

If you are reading this book proactively, without a serious disciplinary order hanging over your head, you may feel even less motivated than these clinicians. Having read this far, you may be tempted to stop here, congratulate yourself on mastering the subject, and shelve the book for future reference.

That would be a terrible shame, because this next section is arguably the most important part of the whole book. It describes the difficult process of gauging your own violation potential and taking concrete steps to reduce it. If you don't think you need to go through all that because you are not in any danger, you are not alone. Virtually all of the disciplined clinicians who are sent to PBI Education remedial courses felt exactly the same way.

Gauging Your Own Violation Potential

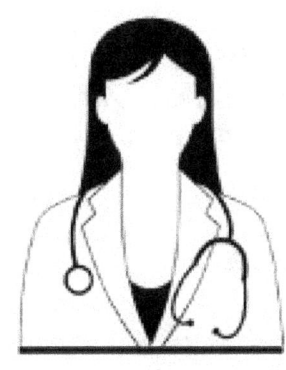

Case File

George, an overweight, sedentary middle-aged physics professor with hypertension and a family history of coronary disease, has just had his annual physical. His physician, Dr. Miller, advises him to avoid extreme exertion, stop smoking, modify his diet, and begin a carefully monitored program of exercise.

When George refuses to believe he is at risk, the doctor cautions him that his heart attack potential, the likelihood of a life-threatening MI, will skyrocket if he doesn't accept her advice. In an effort to reach her patient, Dr. Miller sketches out a "formula:"

$$\text{Heart Attack Potential} = \frac{\text{Risky Behavior} \times \text{Medical Vulnerabilities}}{\text{Rehabilitation Program}} \text{ Resistance to Medical Advice}$$

"Your potential for a heart attack is determined by your medical vulnerabilities (your physical condition, poor health habits, and family history)," she tells him. "Your heart-attack potential increases every time you engage in risky behavior, like sudden exertion, and decreases to the extent you undertake the rehabilitation program I've suggested. Your refusal to confront this situation, your resistance to medical advice, escalates your Heart Attack Potential exponentially.

$$HAP = \left(\frac{R \times M\,Vul}{RP} \right)^R$$

After considering what his doctor has said and written, the patient smiles, picks up a pen and jots down:

"It looks like an equation, but it's impossible to assign numerical values to any of the variables," he laughs. "Yes," replies the physician. "But understanding what it means might well save your life."

The Violation Potential Formula

The Violation Potential Formula does for professional boundaries what Dr. Miller's formula does for coronary disease. Like hers, the VP Formula is not a mathematical equation. You cannot assign numerical values to the variables and compute a precise VP. But once you understand what each of the variables means, you can use the formula to gauge how high your own VP is at any given time, and what steps you need to take to reduce it. *In short, understanding the VP Formula might well save your career.*

$$\text{Violation Potential} = \left(\frac{\text{Risk Factors} \times \text{Vulnerabilities}}{\text{Accountability}} \right)^{\text{Resistance}}$$

Or more succinctly,

$$VP = \left(\frac{RF \times Vul}{A} \right)^{R}$$

Risk Factors

Risk factors are external aspects of your life that are likely to trigger a crossing or violation. Again, some risk factors are common to nearly every clinician—the litigious nature of American culture, the current upheaval in health care reform, the demands of electronic health record keeping, and the opioid epidemic, to name the most obvious. Other risk factors differ from clinician to clinician, such as:

- **Patient population:**

    o   If you practice with either a pediatric or geriatric patient population, the risks of miscommunication are high, both because some patients are unable to communicate with you and because you often have to include multiple family members in your consultations.

    o   As mentioned above, the risk of misunderstandings also increases when your patient has been raised in a culture different from yours.

    o   A critical shortage of psychiatrists means that many psychiatric patients—some of whom are depressed, delusional, or self-destructive—are now being treated by general practitioners who lack adequate mental health training.

- **Type of practice:**
  - If you work in an urban ER, you are exposed to near-constant crises, long hours, and patients you have never seen before and may never see again.
  - In a rural clinic, you are likely to know many of your patients socially, which can blur the boundaries between your professional and personal relationships.
  - Specialties such as ob-gyn, urology, and dermatology involve a steady stream of intimate exams and discussions that can easily be misinterpreted.

- **Types of patients:**
  - Flirtatious patients often seem disarmingly playful, but they are likely to take offense if you respond in kind—or worse, think you're inviting a romantic relationship.
  - Manipulative patients are experts at playing on emotions. They may flatter you, threaten lawsuits, or make you feel guilty. If they succeed, you will do what they want, even if at the risk of a boundary violation.
  - Needy patients seek your attention more than your medical help. They will call with "urgent" problems and seem always to have one more question or symptom. And they tend to react badly if they don't get what they want.

- **Work environment:**
  - Large institutions tend to overlook unprofes-

sional behavior if it helps attract paying patients or financial support. They may even encourage, overtly or otherwise, risky behavior. But they are unlikely to support you if you are charged with a violation.

- ○ Small, intimate practices tend to be casual, which can shrink the "safe space" that boundaries are meant to protect.

- ○ Every workplace has its own culture. Some are supportive and team-based, others are fiercely competitive. Whether or not the culture you work in is a risk factor depends on your particular vulnerabilities.

- **Level of experience:**
  - ○ Inexperienced clinicians just starting out are often unaware of the risks they are taking.
  - ○ Overconfident clinicians, "burdened" by age, wisdom, and experience, often take risks they could easily avoid.
  - ○ Physicians who retire with their license and prescription pad tend to take an overly casual attitude towards treating family and friends.

- **Major life events:**
  - ○ Happy events—a promotion at work, the arrival of a baby, a new house—are exhilarating and apt to embolden risky behavior.
  - ○ Difficult times—caring for aging parents, going through a divorce, suffering the loss of someone close—can be overwhelming and encourage impatience with the demands of professionalism.

o Discipline for a previous violation puts you at heightened risk, because your regulator is now likely to see any new infraction as part of a pattern. Your past magnifies your present.

Vulnerabilities

Vulnerabilities are aspects of your inner life that make you susceptible to particular kinds of boundary violations. Some are unique to you, some are common to just about everyone. Some are transient, others last a lifetime. The most common vulnerabilities include:

- **Physical and mental illness.** Healthcare professionals suffer as much as anyone else from physical and mental health issues, everything from anxiety and chronic pain to addiction and incapacitating injury—all of which interfere with one's ability to take initiative, make good decisions, and respond effectively to stressful situations.

- **Psychological issues.** Unresolved traumas are at the root of many boundary violations. These psychic injuries are often buried well below the level of everyday consciousness, which makes them all the more dangerous. Clinicians make bad decisions and end up crossing boundaries, often without realizing that they are unconsciously seeking to re-enact traumatic experiences from their past.

Over the years, experts have identified certain recurring patterns of vulnerability.

- **People pleasers:** Rather than risk angering or disappointing a patient, "people pleasers" refuse to say "no" or set limits. They will sacrifice their own interests and push themselves further than they know they should in order to avoid losing a patient's good opinion or approval, no matter how unreasonable the person's demands and expectations are.

In their book, *The Wounded Healer,* Richard Irons and Jennifer P. Schneider describe several "archetypes of sexually exploitative males,"[34] some of which can be applied to both men and women who exploit their positions, even in ways unrelated to sex:

- **"The Naïve Prince":** This is a young clinician, flush with power and feeling invulnerable. Professionals in this mold are "suffused with pride." Overconfident and naively unaware of their own emotional needs, these enthusiastic young clinicians rush into challenging situations, whether sexual or not, that they are wholly unprepared for.

- **"The Wounded Warrior":** These clinicians seek to escape inner pain and validate their self-worth by immersing themselves in their work, often neglecting family and friends in the process. For some, this over-commitment is a familiar holdover from training.

- **"The Self-Serving Martyr":** This archetype describes seasoned clinicians who view themselves as pious professionals, willing to sacrifice their own welfare for the benefit of unappreciative patients. Over time, they come to feel

increasingly resentful and may turn to drugs or alcohol to numb the pain.

Risk Factors X Vulnerabilities

The risks you face and your personal vulnerabilities are not simply additive; each magnifies the other. So while it's important to identify both your risk factors and your vulnerabilities, it is even more crucial to think through how they feed off each other.

- A flirtatious patient is always a risk factor, but if you're feeling lonely in the wake of a recent divorce, your vulnerability makes such a patient significantly more dangerous to you.
- If you're in a financial jam, a lucrative business opportunity becomes a serious risk.
- An overbearing supervisor is a risk factor if you have trouble dealing with authority figures.
- Patients and institutions also have vulnerabilities, which can become risk factors for you. The most common institutional vulnerability is the tendency to view patients as customers. (See Part 2.) If you have trouble saying no to patients, hospitals that encourage a "patient-is-always-right" approach will ratchet up your VP.
- Patients' vulnerabilities pose even more of a risk, because you generally don't know about them until it's too late. You only learn about a patient's traumatic childhood of abuse when the gesture you meant to be reassuring comes across as threatening.

Accountability

Most of us learn about accountability first as children, when a parent warns, "I've got my eye on you." The warning itself is often enough to inhibit bad behavior—at least for a time—presumably because we know there will be consequences if we are caught violating the rules. Accountability Theory provides a more sophisticated explanation of essentially the same phenomenon in the adult world. According to the theory, knowing that we may have to justify our actions to a third party leads us to think more seriously about the decisions we make, and therefore, make more responsible choices.

Whichever way you explain it, knowing that someone is watching us—that they will know what we do and judge our performance—seriously decreases our tendency to violate boundaries. The oversight can take many forms, ranging from professional supervision to the mere presence of colleagues or staff nearby. The very act of keeping accurate records, which others will read, is a valuable form of accountability.

Accountability can also be internalized. Just as children learn how to govern their own behavior even when no one is watching, adults govern their behavior based on the norms and ethics they have internalized over the years. Most clinicians, of course, hold themselves accountable in just this way.

It's important to recognize that accountability is a tool you can use to protect yourself and lower your VP. Perhaps the most effective accountability tool, and the most neglected, is the use of chaperones. A chaperone, especially one who is properly trained, provides three layers of accountability. The first is the kind of accountability we've been talking about, the potential need to explain one's actions to another. A second layer is the potential for actual intervention: if a chaperone sees something going wrong, they can step in and stop it. And finally, a chaperone provides objectivity, which helps prevent the kind of "he said, she said" disagreements that often end up before a regulator.

Resistance

It's a lot easier to deny or deflect a problem than it is to confront it. Found guilty of a boundary violation, many clinicians reject the charge, blame the victim, or accuse their regulator of over-reacting. Such resistance prevents constructive action. You can't deal with a problem you refuse to acknowledge.

Overcoming resistance is never easy. But it's especially hard during times of crisis, trauma, transition and loss. When you are already struggling with financial stress or serious health issues, the last thing you want to do is start wrestling with still more troubling problems. Rather than facing up to your demons at such times, you are more likely to simply deny that you have turned your back on them.

A provider in denial may refuse to take responsibility for an angry outburst by blaming it on the patient's "outrageous behavior." But when they refuse to accept that blaming the victim is just a form of resistance, a way of avoiding the painful reality of their own behavior, they wall themself off from even considering the possibility that they are at fault. They are in the throes of double-R, resisting awareness of their own resistance, expressed in the formula as R^R.

$$\text{Violation Potential} = \left(\frac{\text{Risk Factors} \times \text{Vulnerabilities}}{\text{Accountability}} \right)^{R^{R}}$$

Or

$$VP = \left(\frac{RF \times Vul}{A} \right)^{R^{R^R}}$$

Catalyst

Even if you have a high VP, you may well avoid a violation until a catalyst ignites the explosive mixture of resistance, vulnerabilities, risk factors and accountability represented by the Violation Potential Formula. A catalyst can be anything—a patient who pushes your buttons, a crisis at work or home—depending on your particular situation.

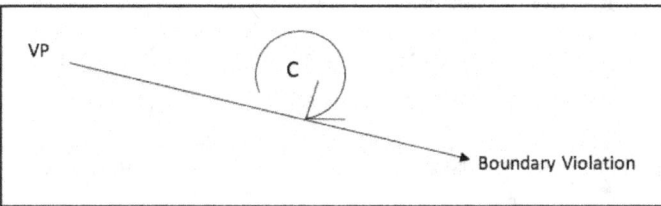

Putting The Formula To Work

It's one thing to understand the Violation Potential Formula. Putting it to work, using honest assessments of your own situation, is something else entirely. It is difficult, if not impossible, to do by yourself. If you have a colleague or partner who knows you well, ask for their help. Their job is to keep you honest, prevent you from ducking tough issues, and encourage you when you start to falter. If they do their job well, you will probably get defensive and begin to wish you had never started the process. Hang in there, and remember that the discomfort you are feeling is nothing compared to the pain you are working to avoid.

And don't forget the second half of Law #1: *Everyone has a violation potential,* **and it is constantly changing.** Whenever your situation changes significantly, take some time to consider how it affects your VP.

To illustrate how the VP formula works, we will be looking at the vulnerabilities, risk factors, resistance and accountability of three different clinicians: doctors Blue, Green and Brown.

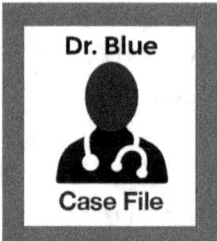

Dr. Blue is a 32-year-old chiropractor, working at a large, multi-specialty practice. It is her first full-time position and some of the staff has teased her about being "wet behind the ears." She wants to be a good sport, but is eager to prove herself a skilled and reliable clinician.

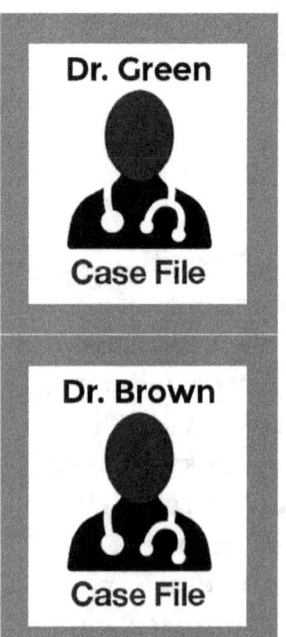

Dr. Green is a 40-year old orthopedist with two young children and a third on the way. He was recently promoted to a tenured spot in the medical school of the university where he works and has a full panel of patients.

Dr. Brown is the senior partner in a dental practice that he started nearly 20 years ago. His three children are in college and graduate school, and his wife, an environmental engineer, travels frequently to deliver papers and consult overseas.

Coming To Terms With Your Vulnerabilities

Reminder: Vulnerabilities are aspects of your inner life that make you susceptible to particular kinds of boundary violations.

As you begin to brainstorm vulnerabilities, consider things that keep you up at night or worry you during the day. Recurring fantasies of escape and daydreams of

triumph can help point you towards less obvious insecurities and fears.

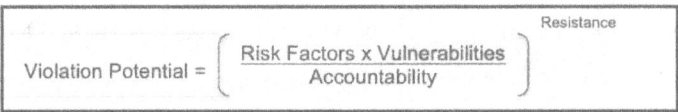

Other vulnerabilities may be lurking in the shadows, but they can be nudged into the daylight with a little persistence. Below is a checklist to help get you started. Hopefully, as you work through it—ideally with someone you trust—you will probably begin to notice concerns and challenges of your own that aren't on the list.

This is not a one-and-done process and need not be time-consuming. The goal is not to create an exhaustive list and move on, but to develop a habit of mind that helps you take note of vulnerabilities as they occur to you throughout your career. *Tip: Be sure to watch for red flag moments.*

Overcoming resistance.

As you work to identify vulnerabilities, you will almost certainly have to contend with resistance. It can take many forms—anger, denial, diversion ("my problem isn't impatience, it's that incompetent assistant"). Before you reject the possibility of a vulnerability, take a step back and consider whether you might be trying to avoid a genuine issue. Once again, a third party can provide valuable feedback here.

Identifying Vulnerabilities: A partial checklist

- **Personal concerns** — Do you feel unappreciated, overwhelmed, resentful?

- **Family concerns** — Are you having marital problems, or worried about kids or aging parents?

- **Professional concerns** — Do you have challenging supervisors, difficult patients, or career concerns?

- **Social concerns** — Do you lack close friends? Do you feel isolated or lonely?

- **Stage of life** — Do you feel burdened by too much responsibility? Are you questioning the choices you've made? Are you worried about empty-nesting or retiring?

- **Financial stress** — Are you worried about student debt, paying for college, or saving for retirement?

- **Emotional distress** — Are you experiencing grief, guilt, anger, depression, or anxiety—with or without obvious causes?

- **Physical distress** — Is chronic pain or illness interfering with your personal or professional life?

- **Mental distress** — Are you having trouble focusing? Are you having obsessive thoughts?

> ***Dr. Blue*** *remembers a colleague urging her to be less defensive. "You keep reacting to well-meaning guidance*

THE PHYSICIAN'S GUIDE TO PROFESSIONAL BOUNDARIES

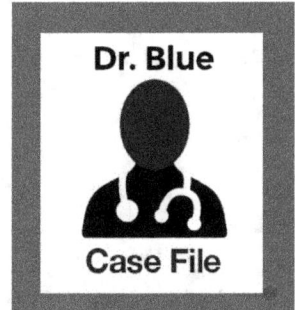

as if it was unfair criticism." She laughed off the advice at the time, but has since noticed how defensive she gets when others offer suggestions. After snapping at an experienced nurse for offering advice, she realized how bullheaded she was being and apologized.

Vulnerabilities: Insecurity about her lack of experience, over-sensitive to criticism, headstrong

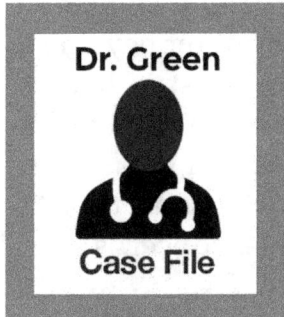

Dr. Green frequently recalls how his father, also a physician, used to spend time with patients in his home office and still join the family for dinner every night. When he mentioned his memory to his mother, she laughed and said things were never that tranquil. As he thought about it, he realized how rushed he felt with patients and how much he missed spending time with his young family. **Vulnerabilities:** Feeling rushed and emotionally deprived

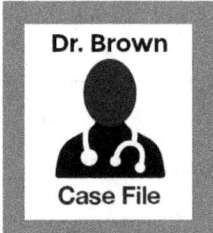

Dr. Brown was about to reprimand a young dentist in his practice for being too chummy with patients when he realized he was guilty of exactly the same offense. He had recently been sharing stories about his kids with patients and talking with several women about their social lives. As he thought about where this was coming *from and where it might take him, he realized he had some pretty serious vulnerabilities.* **Vulnerabilities:** *Lonely, missing kids away at school and wife away for work*

Identifying Your Risk Factors

Reminder: Risk factors are external aspects of your life that are likely to trigger a crossing or violation.

A risk factor may be harmless in one situation and perilous in another. Once you identify a concern, it's important to consider when it is likely to cause a problem. Some of this is common sense. If you are worried about money, the patient who is constantly inviting you to invest in business schemes is clearly a risk factor. Other risks will likely occur to you once you are sensitized to your vulnerability. When your kids complain that you never play with them anymore, you may realize how your financial concerns are pushing you to work late into the night.

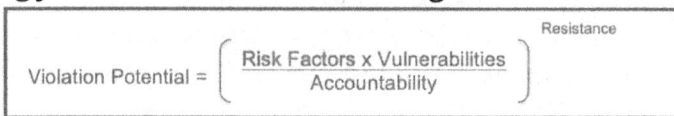

Other risk factors are independent of your particular vulnerabilities. If many of your patients are recent immigrants, cultural issues should definitely be on your radar. But keep in mind that risks and vulnerabilities often magnify each other. You might have considered your ability to defuse tension with humor a strength rather than a vulnerability, but a patient from a different culture may not get the joke and take offense. When interacting with such patients your strength becomes a vulnerability.

Tip: In light of your vulnerabilities and risk factors, consider what kinds of catalysts are likely to spark a violation. If one of your vulnerabilities is a craving for affection, working with a reassuring colleague you find attractive is a risk factor. Attending an out-of-town conference with the same person might well catalyze a violation.

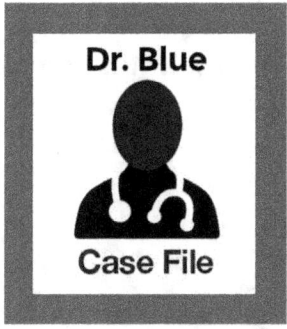

When Dr. Blue complained about the "insufferable old-school blowhard" supervising her, a friend said, "Wow! Where did that come from? You were always the understanding one back in chiropractor school." It made Dr. Blue realize how the older domineering doctor triggered her defensiveness.

- **Vulnerabilities:** Over-sensitive to criticism, headstrong
  - **Risk Factor:** Domineering supervisor
    - **Potential Catalyst:** Serious criticism by supervisor

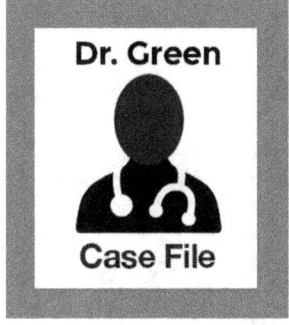

Many of Dr. Green's patients are elderly. Now that he realizes how rushed he feels, he recognizes how exasperated he sometimes gets with slower moving patients. He finds those who are also emotionally needy particularly annoying, the result he suspects of his own depleted emotional reserves. A pileup of such patients might just push him off the edge.

- **Vulnerabilities:** Feeling rushed and emotionally deprived
  - **Risk Factor:** Needy elderly patients
    - **Potential Catalyst:** Pileup of needy patients

Dr. Brown quickly recognizes that female patients who are warm and friendly are a definite risk factor for him, especially those who are emotionally needy themselves. While he always has a dental hygienist or assistant pre-

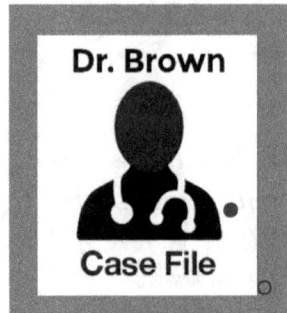

sent, his discussions with patients afterward are one-on-one. When he catches himself fantasizing about a patient named Jenna, he knows he's found a potential catalyst,

Vulnerabilities: *Lonely, missing kids and wife*

Risk Factors: *Supportive, needy patients; unchaperoned consultations*

■ **Potential Catalyst:** *Private consultations with Jenna*

Lowering Your Vp By Increasing Accountability

Reminder: Knowing you are being held accountable encourages more responsible choices.

Consider what kinds of accountability are currently in place at work, and honestly assess how much each influences your decisions and behavior.

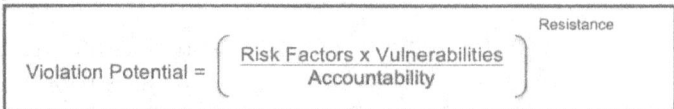

$$\text{Violation Potential} = \left(\frac{\text{Risk Factors} \times \text{Vulnerabilities}}{\text{Accountability}} \right)^{\text{Resistance}}$$

- If you use a chaperone, how likely are they to confront you if necessary?

- If you regularly review cases with a supervisor, how honest are you about potential boundary issues, and how seriously would your supervisor take such concerns?

- Do you include boundary concerns in your notes? If not, ask yourself why you don't.

- How well do you hold yourself accountable? Do you admit mistakes or near-misses to anyone else? To yourself?

Dr. Blue's main source of accountability is also her pri-

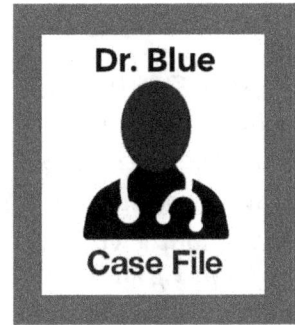

mary risk factor: her domineering supervisor. Unless she looks for another job, she has to find a way to resolve this conflict. Since uninvited criticism angers her, she decides to actively invite it. She tells her supervisor she is eager to improve and asks if rather than offering advice on the fly, he would be willing to meet regularly for an honest critique of her work.

- **Vulnerabilities:** Over-sensitive to criticism, headstrong
  - **Risk Factor:** Domineering supervisor
    - **Potential Catalyst:** Serious criticism by supervisor
      - **Accountability:** Regular critiques with supervisor

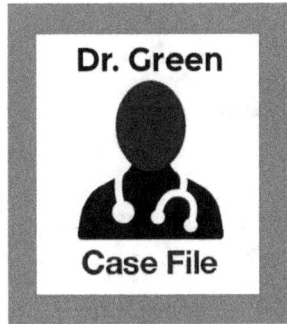

Dr. Green decides to increase his accountability in two ways. First, he is going to share his concerns with his office manager and ask to review daily schedules with him to help identify potential pile-ups ahead of time. He is also going to hire a medical scribe to take notes, which will help lighten his load and provide a chaperone of sorts who can alert him to any problems early on.

- **Vulnerabilities:** Feeling rushed and emotionally deprived
  - **Risk Factor:** Needy elderly patients
    - **Potential Catalyst:** Pileup of needy patients
      - **Accountability:** Review schedules with office manager; hire a scribe/chaperone

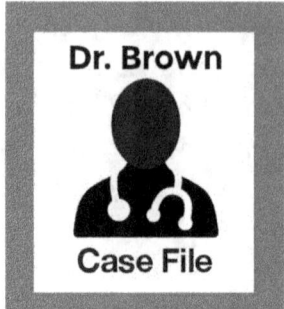

Dr. Brown decides on two strategies to reduce his VP. The first is to make sure a member of his staff is present at all times. The second is to talk to his wife about how he is feeling and his concerns about work, particularly Jenna. He's not sure how his wife will react, but he thinks reconnecting honestly with her is important both for his career and his marriage.

- **Vulnerabilities:** Lonely, missing kids and wife
  - **Risk Factors:** Supportive, needy patients; unchaperoned consultations
    - **Potential Catalyst:** Private consultations with Jenna
    - **Accountability:** Use a chaperone; talk to his wife

Creating A Protection Plan

My Protection Plan

My Vulnerabilities:
My Risk Factors:
My Plan:

Organizational: Changes you will make to office policies, staffing, culture...

Professional: How you plan to manage yourself at work...

Personal: How you plan to ensure a healthy work-life balance...

There are several reasons to create a written protection plan like the one shown here. The simple act of writing down what you've learned about your violation potential and how you plan to reduce it helps fix the plan in your mind. The written record also provides another layer of accountability, as long as you regularly check to see if you are in fact doing what you said you would do.

Tip: To maximize accountability, share your plan with someone else and review it regularly with them.

Another key value of a written plan is that it enables you to consider how things have changed. Some vulnerabilities are likely to dissipate as new ones emerge. New situations will alter your risk factors, suggesting new ways of increasing your accountability. Any time you realize something significant has changed, take out your plan and review it.

The formal structure of the plan also ensures that you consider all the ways you might lower your VP, organizationally, personally, and professionally.

Organizationally. Think through how changing the logistics at work might help.

- Are there tasks that are being slighted or even ignored?
- Would new or different staff members help?
- Is your current staff well-trained and equipped to do their jobs well?
- Can office procedures be tweaked to relieve stress points?
- Can new or revised policies help address issues you've identified as causes for concern?
- How helpful or harmful is the current office culture?

Professionally. What do you need to do differently at work to lower your VP?

- How can you minimize the risk of dual relationships?
- Are any work habits compounding potential problems?
- Should you be using a scribe or chaperone?
- Are there tasks you can delegate?
- Are there professional relationships you are neglecting or others you should scale back?
- Would it be helpful to get more feedback from patients and/or staff?

- Are you well supervised?
- Do you feel competent to manage challenges or would education or mentoring be helpful?

Personally. How can you lessen your vulnerabilities and strengthen your personal wellbeing?

- How can you improve your work-life balance?
- How can you improve your physical and mental health?
- How will you strengthen personal relationships?
- How will you carve out time for yourself?
- How will you enrich your life outside of work?

Takeaways

$$\text{Violation Potential} = \left(\frac{\text{Risk Factors} \times \text{Vulnerabilities}}{\text{Accountability}} \right) \begin{array}{l} \text{Resistance} \\ \text{Resistance} \end{array}$$

- Vulnerabilities are aspects of your inner life that make you susceptible to boundary violations. Psychological issues, both known and unrecognized, are often the most dangerous.

- Risk Factors are external aspects of your life that are likely to trigger a crossing or violation. Common risks include types of patients, work environment, and stressful times of life.

- Risks and vulnerabilities are not simply additive; each magnifies the other.

- Knowing you are being held accountable by others encourages more responsible choices.

- Keeping accurate records that others may read is a valuable

THE PHYSICIAN'S GUIDE TO PROFESSIONAL BOUNDARIES

form of accountability.

- Refusing to acknowledge problems (i.e., "resistance") increases VP exponentially. Double resistance, refusing to acknowledge your resistance, compounds the danger.

- Accountability is a tool you can use to protect yourself and lower your VP. Chaperones are an important and often neglected source of accountability.

- Gauging your own VP means honestly assessing your vulnerabilities, risk factors, resistance, and accountability. This is nearly impossible to do on your own.

- Creating a written protection plan increases accountability and encourages regular reviews. Following an established format ensures that you consider all aspects of your situation.

AFTERWORD

Health care has changed more in the past 50 years than it has in the preceding 2,000. People have not. Hippocrates would surely marvel at x-rays and MRIs, antibiotics and vaccines, but I'm pretty sure he would find the personal and professional challenges you've been reading about all too familiar. The simple sacred oath he wrote is, after all, the first known description of professional boundaries.

Over the years, we have come to understand more about the destabilizing forces that push clinicians past these boundaries and I'd like to think we have put the knowledge to good use, helping those who have made mistakes recover. The greater challenge is helping others avoid the same mistakes in the first place.

Pain is a great motivator. As I mentioned earlier, many individuals find the strength to make needed changes only after they have endured the pain of serious discipline. But you don't have to learn the hard way. For all our flaws, we human beings have a rare capacity to learn not just from our own mistakes but also from each other. The same empathy that helps you understand what your patients are going through can help you understand what your colleagues have suffered. By identifying with them you give yourself a chance to learn from their pain rather than your own.

You will be tempted to distance yourself from these colleagues—from the "cases" you have read about in this book—to tell yourself you would never make such mistakes. Do yourself a favor and recognize this impulse for what it is: Resistance. Instead, consider your own vulnerabilities and risk factors, and do what you can to increase your accountability. As I said at the outset, think of this book as preventive medicine.

Remember, your license to practice is not a right you are entitled to. It is a rare and precious privilege you have been entrusted with. Treasure it and protect it at all times.

—Dr. Stephen Schenthal, CEO,
PBI Education

ENDNOTES

[1] Strasburger L. Practical boundary keeping. Primary Psychiatry. http://primarypsychiatry.com/practical-boundary-keeping/. April 1, 2002. Accessed May 18, 2019.

[2] Peterson MR. At Personal Risk. New York: W.W. Norton & Company; 1992: 47.

[3] Practitioner's Manual - SECTION V: Valid Prescription Requirements. U.S. Department of Justice, Drug Enforcement Division. https://www.deadiversion.usdoj.gov/pubs/manuals/pract/section5.htm. Accessed on May 21, 2019

[4] Adapted from: Prescription drug epidemic: 20 red flags physicians should watch for. The DO. June 11, 2015. https://thedo.osteopathic.org/2015/06/prescription-drug-epidemic-20-red-flags-physicians-should-watch-for/ Accessed May 21, 2019

[5] U.S. Medical Regulatory Trends and Actions 2018. Federation of State Medical Boards — How State Medical Boards Share Information about Disciplined Physicians. 2018. https://www.fsmb.org/siteassets/advocacy/publications/us-medical-regulatory-trends-actions.pdf, Accessed May 31, 2019

[6] Graber MA. Treating friends poses both risks and compromises. American Medical News. https://amednews.com/article/20110606/profession/306069945/5/. June 6, 2011. Accessed May 18, 2019.

[7] American Medical Association. Code of Medical Ethics. https://www.ama-assn.org/sites/ama-assn.org/files/corp/media-browser/principles-of-medical-ethics.pdf. Accessed May 19, 2019.

[8] American College of Physicians. Ethics Manual. https://

www.acponline.org/clinical-information/ethics-and-professionalism/acp-ethics-manual-seventh-edition-a-comprehensive-medical-ethics-resource/acp-ethics-manual-seventh-edition. Accessed May 18, 2019.

[9] Arshack DN, Knight DJ. It's Just Not OK: Sexual Relations Between Physicians and their Patients. New York Law Journal, March 7, 2013;Vol. 249(44):4-6.

[10] "The National Practitioner Data Bank (NPDB) is a web-based repository of reports containing information on medical malpractice payments and certain adverse actions related to health care practitioners, providers, and suppliers. Established by Congress in 1986, it is a workforce tool that prevents practitioners from moving state to state without disclosure or discovery of previous damaging performance." U.S. Department of Health and Human Services, NPDP, About Us. https://www.npdb.hrsa.gov/topNavigation/aboutUs.jsp. Accessed May 31, 2019.

[11] Hughes D. Medical students set bad example by doctors, says research. BBC News. https://www.bbc.com/news/health-23072562. July 1, 2013. Accessed May 18, 2019.

[12] Roy v. Medical Board of California, Real Party in Interest. https://caselaw.findlaw.com/ca-court-of-appeal/1460907.html. Accessed May 18, 2019.

[13] To empathize or not to empathize. PBI Education Blog. https://pbieducation.com/to-empathize-or-not-to-empathize/. Accessed May 20, 2019.

[14] Pronovost PJ. Learning Accountability for Patient Outcomes. JAMA. 2010;304(2):204–205.

[15] Peterson, p. 60-61.

[16] Nimmon L, Stenfors-Hayes T. The 'Handling' of power in the physician-patient encounter: perceptions from experienced physicians. BMC Medical Education. https://docs.google.com/document/d/1vlDGaJWgxJSlVui2g-wXKEuI0cbG2xGpgFdztersskEU/edit#. Accessed May 18, 2019.

[17] The Practical Professional, Issue 18, October/November 2018

[18] Ibid.

[19] Yale Perception and Cognition Laboratory. Reference Guide: Inattentional Blindness. http://perception.yale.edu/Brian/refGuides/IB.html. Updated 8/11/17. Accessed May 19, 2019.

[20] Chabrism C, Simons D. The Invisible Gorilla. New York. Crown; 2010: 22.

[21] Competency and retirement: Evaluating the senior physician. American Medical Association. https://www.ama-assn.org/practice-management/physician-diversity/competency-and-retirement-evaluating-senior-physician. Accessed May 19, 2019.

[22] Medscape National Physician Burnout & Depression Report 2018. https://www.medscape.com/slideshow/2018-lifestyle-burnout-depression-6009235. Accessed May 19, 2019.

[23] Gerada C. For doctors with mental illness, 'help me' can be the hardest words. The Guardian. https://www.theguardian.com/commentisfree/2018/jun/06/doctors-mental-health-problems-taboo. June 6, 2018. Accessed May 19, 2019.

[24] Dahle JM. Physicians are financially illiterate and it's time for that to change. KevinMD.com. https://www.kevinmd.com/blog/2017/03/physicians-financially-illiterate-time-change.html. March 21, 2017. Accessed May 19, 2019.

[25] The Practical Professional, Issue 9, December/January 2017

[26] Solon O. Compassion over empathy could help prevent emotional burnout. Wired.com. https://www.wired.co.uk/article/tania-singer-compassion-burnout. Accessed May 21, 2019

[27] Dusquesne University School of Nursing. Delivering Culturally Competent Care. Duquesne University School of Nurs-

ing. https://onlinenursing.duq.edu/blog/delivering-culturally-competent-care/. Accessed May 19, 2019.

[28] A Roadmap for New Physicians, I. Physician Relationships With Payers. Office of Inspector General Department of Health and Human Services. https://oig.hhs.gov/compliance/physician-education/02payers.asp. Accessed May 19, 2019.

[29] American Medical Association. Code of Medical Ethics, Opinion 9.1.1.

[30] American Psychological Association. Ethical Principles of Psychologists and Code of Conduct, 10.08 Sexual Intimacies with former therapy clients/patients. https://www.apa.org/ethics/code/. Accessed May 19, 2019.

[31] Greyson SR. Physician Violations of Online Professionalism and Disciplinary Actions: A National Survey of State Medical Boards. Jamanetwork.com. March 1, 2012. Accessed May 21, 2019. https://jamanetwork.com/journals/jama/fullarticle/1105088

[32] California Court of Appeal. Roy v. Superior Court (Med. Bd. of California) https://caselaw.findlaw.com/summary/opinion/ca-court-of-appeal/2011/08/31/256228.html. Accessed May 19, 2019.

[33] Greene A. HIPAA compliance for clinician texting. American Health Information Management Association. http://bok.ahima.org/doc?oid=105342#.XOHoDchKjDY. Accessed May 19, 2019.

[34] Irons R., Schneider JP. The Wounded Healer: Addiction-Sensitive Approach to the Sexually Exploitative Professional. New York: Jason Aronson, Inc.; 1977.

www.ingramcontent.com/pod-product-compliance
Lightning Source LLC
Chambersburg PA
CBHW050000230526
45465CB00003BB/1195